Flat Belly Anti-Inflammatory Diet for Beginners 2025

Easy and Budget-Friendly Ways to Minimize Bloating, Enhance Digestive Health, and Promote Optimal wellbeing

Aaron F. Nolan

Copyright © 2024 Don Frank. All rights reserved.

No part of this book may be reproduced, distributed, or transmitted in any form or by any means, including photocopying, recording, or other electronic or mechanical methods, without the prior written permission of the publisher, except in the case of brief quotations embodied in critical reviews and certain other non-commercial uses permitted by copyright law.

Disclaimer: The information contained in this book is for educational and informational purposes only. The author and publisher make no representations or warranties with respect to the accuracy or completeness of the contents. The advice and strategies contained herein may not be suitable for your situation. You should consult with a professional where appropriate.

Any references to historical events, real people, or real places are used fictitiously. Other names, characters, places, and events are products of the author's imagination, and any resemblance to actual events, locales, or persons, living or dead, is entirely coincidental.

Table of Content

Introduction 4

    What is Inflammation and Why It Matters 4

    How Inflammation Affects Belly Fat 4

    The Science Behind the Flat Belly Anti-Inflammatory Diet 5

    Benefits of an Anti-Inflammatory Lifestyle 5

    How to Use This Cookbook 5

    Essential Anti-Inflammatory Ingredients & Pantry Staples 6

        Tools and Equipment You'll Need 6

        Tips for Meal Planning and Prep 6

Breakfasts to Start Your Day Right 7

Energizing Snacks & Small Bites 24

Light & Refreshing Salads 46

Satisfying Soups & Stews 70

Wholesome Main Courses 94

Side Dishes Packed With Flavor 118

30-Day Anti-Inflammatory Meal Plan 141

Conclusion 146

Introduction

Welcome to *"Flat Belly Anti-Inflammatory Diet for Beginners 2025,"* your essential guide to achieving a healthier, leaner body by harnessing the power of anti-inflammatory foods. If you're tired of endless diets that don't deliver long-lasting results, or you feel bloated and sluggish despite your best efforts, then this book is for you.

Inflammation is a natural process in your body, meant to defend against infection or injury. However, when inflammation becomes chronic, it wreaks havoc on your system, contributing to weight gain, particularly around the belly, as well as numerous chronic diseases. The good news is that by adopting an anti-inflammatory diet, you can not only reduce belly fat but also improve your overall well-being. This guide will show you how to do just that, step by step.

What is Inflammation and Why It Matters

Inflammation plays a vital role in the body's immune response, but when it becomes persistent, it can lead to a range of health problems such as heart disease, diabetes, and obesity. These chronic conditions are often linked to unhealthy lifestyle choices, particularly diet. Certain foods, like processed sugars, trans fats, and refined carbs, can trigger inflammatory responses in the body, leading to excess weight gain, especially around the midsection.

This book focuses on introducing foods and recipes that fight inflammation, promote gut health, and balance your body's internal systems. The result? A flatter belly, enhanced energy levels, and improved mental clarity.

How Inflammation Affects Belly Fat

The connection between inflammation and belly fat is often underestimated. Chronic inflammation disrupts the body's hormonal balance, particularly insulin and cortisol levels, which are key players in fat storage. When your body is constantly inflamed, it holds onto fat, making it harder to lose weight—even with exercise. By targeting inflammation at its source, you're not just shedding pounds; you're actively healing your body from within.

The Science Behind the Flat Belly Anti-Inflammatory Diet

This diet is grounded in research on foods that naturally reduce inflammation, stabilize blood sugar, and promote fat loss. You'll learn how simple dietary changes can have profound impacts on your body's inflammation levels. From antioxidant-rich fruits and vegetables to omega-3 packed fish and nuts, each recipe in this book is designed to soothe inflammation while supporting fat metabolism and digestion.

Benefits of an Anti-Inflammatory Lifestyle

Beyond weight loss, the benefits of an anti-inflammatory lifestyle are immense. Reduced inflammation helps lower the risk of chronic diseases, improves joint health, boosts your immune system, and enhances skin complexion. Not to mention, you'll feel more energized, sleep better, and experience fewer digestive issues.

How to Use This Cookbook

Whether you're new to the anti-inflammatory diet or looking to deepen your knowledge, this cookbook is your comprehensive resource. Each recipe is crafted with nutrient-dense, anti-inflammatory ingredients that are easy to find and simple to prepare. You'll find meal options for every part of the day—whether it's a quick breakfast, a wholesome lunch, a satisfying dinner, or even a guilt-free dessert.

Start with the recipes that fit your daily routine, or dive into meal planning with the provided tips for batch cooking and organizing your pantry. This book is flexible enough to support your unique lifestyle while ensuring you stay on track with your goals.

Essential Anti-Inflammatory Ingredients & Pantry Staples

To make this journey easier, we've included a guide to must-have ingredients and pantry staples that will become your go-to items. Think turmeric, ginger, leafy greens, wild-caught salmon, berries, and nuts. Stocking your kitchen with these anti-inflammatory powerhouses will make it effortless to whip up healthy, delicious meals any time of day.

Tools and Equipment You'll Need

No complicated gadgets or pricey tools are necessary! We've kept it simple, focusing on basic kitchen essentials you likely already own, like a good chef's knife, blender, and cast-iron skillet. These tools will help you prepare the recipes quickly and efficiently.

Tips for Meal Planning and Prep

Success in any diet comes down to preparation. We'll guide you through meal planning strategies to ensure you stay ahead of the game, even with a busy schedule. From batch-cooking grains to prepping veggies in advance, these tips will save you time and effort, making your anti-inflammatory journey as stress-free as possible.

By the end of this book, you'll have a deep understanding of how the foods you eat can either fuel inflammation or fight it, and more importantly, how to make choices that will leave you feeling and looking your best.

Let's get started on the journey toward a healthier, happier you—one delicious, anti-inflammatory meal at a time!

Chapter 1

Breakfasts to Start Your Day Right

Turmeric Scrambled Tofu with Spinach

This recipe for *Turmeric Scrambled Tofu with Spinach* is a nutrient-packed, anti-inflammatory alternative to traditional scrambled eggs. It's loaded with plant-based protein, anti-inflammatory turmeric, and leafy greens, making it a fantastic choice for a nourishing breakfast or brunch. The combination of tofu and spinach creates a delicious, savory dish that not only satisfies your taste buds but also helps combat inflammation, leaving you energized and ready to start your day.

Preparation Time

- **Prep Time**: 10 minutes
- **Cook Time**: 10 minutes
- **Total Time**: 20 minutes

Ingredients

- 1 block (14 oz) firm or extra-firm tofu, drained and crumbled
- 2 cups fresh spinach, chopped
- 1 small onion, finely chopped
- 1 clove garlic, minced
- 1 tablespoon olive oil
- 1 teaspoon ground turmeric
- ½ teaspoon ground cumin
- ¼ teaspoon smoked paprika (optional)
- Salt and pepper to taste
- 1 tablespoon nutritional yeast (optional, for cheesy flavor)
- 1 tablespoon lemon juice (optional, for a zesty finish)
- Fresh herbs (like parsley or cilantro) for garnish

Procedure

1. **Prepare the Tofu**: Drain and press the tofu to remove excess water. Once drained, crumble the tofu with your hands or a fork to create a texture similar to scrambled eggs. Set aside.

2. **Sauté the Aromatics**: Heat olive oil in a large skillet over medium heat. Add the chopped onion and cook until translucent, about 3 minutes. Add the minced garlic and sauté for another minute until fragrant.

3. **Season the Tofu**: Add the crumbled tofu to the skillet and stir in the turmeric, cumin, and smoked paprika (if using). These spices will give the tofu a beautiful golden color and add anti-inflammatory benefits, especially from the turmeric. Stir everything together until the tofu is evenly coated.

4. **Cook the Tofu**: Cook the tofu for 5–7 minutes, stirring occasionally, until it starts to become lightly crispy on the edges. If the tofu looks dry, you can add a splash of water or vegetable broth to keep it moist.

5. **Add the Spinach**: Once the tofu is cooked, stir in the chopped spinach. Cook for another 2–3 minutes until the spinach is wilted and tender.

6. **Enhance the Flavor**: Stir in the nutritional yeast for a cheesy flavor (optional), and add lemon juice for a zesty kick. Season with salt and pepper to taste.

7. **Serve**: Remove from heat and garnish with fresh herbs like parsley or cilantro. Serve hot as is, or pair with whole-grain toast or a side of avocado for a more filling meal.

Nutritional Value (per serving)

- **Calories**: ~200
- **Protein**: 15g
- **Carbohydrates**: 8g
- **Fiber**: 4g
- **Fat**: 12g
- **Saturated Fat**: 2g
- **Sodium**: 250mg
- **Vitamin A**: 50% of daily recommended intake
- **Vitamin C**: 20% of daily recommended intake

- **Calcium**: 15% of daily recommended intake
- **Iron**: 25% of daily recommended intake

This *Turmeric Scrambled Tofu with Spinach* is not only packed with protein but also rich in vitamins and minerals, particularly iron, calcium, and antioxidants from the spinach and turmeric. It's a quick and easy meal, perfect for anyone following an anti-inflammatory diet. You can adjust the spices to your liking or add more vegetables for extra nutrition.

Blueberry Chia Pudding

Blueberry Chia Pudding is a delicious, nutritious, and anti-inflammatory breakfast or snack that's packed with fiber, omega-3 fatty acids, and antioxidants. The chia seeds, known for their ability to absorb liquid and form a gel-like consistency, create a thick, creamy pudding base without any need for cooking. Combined with blueberries, which are high in anti-inflammatory phytonutrients, this pudding makes for a powerhouse of nutrients that support gut health, reduce inflammation, and boost overall energy levels.

Preparation Time

- **Prep Time**: 5 minutes
- **Chill Time**: 4 hours (or overnight)
- **Total Time**: 4 hours 5 minutes

Ingredients

- 1/4 cup chia seeds
- 1 cup unsweetened almond milk (or any plant-based milk)
- 1/2 cup fresh or frozen blueberries
- 1 tablespoon maple syrup (or honey, optional)
- 1/2 teaspoon vanilla extract
- 1 tablespoon almond butter (optional, for extra creaminess)
- 1 tablespoon lemon juice (optional, to enhance the blueberry flavor)

- Fresh blueberries and mint leaves for garnish

Procedure

1. **Combine Chia Seeds and Liquid**: In a medium-sized bowl or jar, add the chia seeds and unsweetened almond milk. Stir well to ensure the seeds are evenly distributed and no clumps form.
2. **Add Sweeteners and Flavorings**: Stir in the maple syrup (or honey, if using), vanilla extract, and almond butter for extra creaminess. These ingredients add natural sweetness and enhance the flavor of the pudding. If you prefer a zesty touch, mix in the lemon juice.
3. **Blend the Blueberries**: In a blender, puree the 1/2 cup of blueberries until smooth. If you want a chunkier texture, you can mash them with a fork instead of blending.
4. **Mix in the Blueberries**: Stir the blueberry puree into the chia mixture, ensuring the blueberries are fully incorporated. This will give the pudding its beautiful purple hue and a burst of berry flavor.
5. **Chill the Pudding**: Cover the bowl or jar with a lid or plastic wrap, and place it in the refrigerator to set for at least 4 hours, or preferably overnight. The chia seeds will absorb the liquid and thicken the pudding.
6. **Stir Before Serving**: Before serving, give the pudding a good stir to break up any clumps and check the consistency. If it's too thick, you can add a little more almond milk to loosen it up.
7. **Serve and Garnish**: Serve the chia pudding in small bowls or jars, and top with fresh blueberries, a drizzle of maple syrup, and a few mint leaves for garnish.

Avocado Toast with Hemp Seeds & Microgreens is a simple yet nutrient-dense meal that can be enjoyed for breakfast, lunch, or a snack. This dish combines the creamy richness of avocado, the nutty flavor of hemp seeds, and the fresh crunch of microgreens, creating a balanced and flavorful meal that's rich in healthy fats, fiber, and essential nutrients. Avocados are well-known for their heart-healthy monounsaturated fats and anti-inflammatory properties, while hemp seeds provide plant-based protein and omega-3 fatty acids. Microgreens add a fresh burst of vitamins and minerals, making this an easy-to-make, anti-inflammatory recipe that's as delicious as it is nutritious.

Preparation Time

- **Prep Time**: 5 minutes
- **Cook Time**: 5 minutes
- **Total Time**: 10 minutes

Ingredients

- 2 slices of whole-grain or sourdough bread
- 1 ripe avocado
- 1 tablespoon hemp seeds
- 1/2 cup microgreens (such as arugula, kale, or radish)
- 1 teaspoon lemon juice
- 1 tablespoon extra virgin olive oil (optional)
- Salt and pepper to taste
- Red pepper flakes or chili flakes (optional, for a kick of heat)

Procedure

1. **Toast the Bread**: Begin by toasting the whole-grain or sourdough bread slices until they are golden and crisp. You can use a toaster or a stovetop grill pan to achieve the desired crunch.

2. **Prepare the Avocado**: While the bread is toasting, cut the avocado in half, remove the pit, and scoop the flesh into a small bowl. Mash the avocado with a fork until smooth but still slightly chunky.

3. **Season the Avocado**: Add the lemon juice to the mashed avocado to enhance its flavor and prevent it from browning. Drizzle in the extra virgin olive oil (optional) for a smoother texture. Season with salt and pepper to taste, and mix well.

4. **Spread the Avocado**: Once the bread is toasted, spread the mashed avocado evenly onto each slice, creating a thick, creamy layer that covers the entire surface.

5. **Sprinkle with Hemp Seeds**: Sprinkle the hemp seeds generously over the avocado spread. Hemp seeds provide a nutty flavor and a boost of protein and omega-3s, making this toast even more nutritious.

6. **Add the Microgreens**: Top the avocado toast with a handful of fresh microgreens. Microgreens not only add a beautiful color contrast but also provide an extra dose of vitamins, minerals, and antioxidants.

7. **Finish and Serve**: If you like a little heat, sprinkle some red pepper flakes or chili flakes on top. Serve immediately, and enjoy the fresh, flavorful combination of avocado, hemp seeds, and microgreens.

Nutritional Value (per serving)

- **Calories**: ~320
- **Protein**: 8g
- **Carbohydrates**: 26g
- **Fiber**: 9g
- **Fat**: 24g
  - **Saturated Fat**: 3.5g
- **Sodium**: 200mg
- **Potassium**: 650mg
- **Vitamin A**: 20% of daily recommended intake
- **Vitamin C**: 25% of daily recommended intake
- **Calcium**: 6% of daily recommended intake
- **Iron**: 10% of daily recommended intake

Avocado Toast with Hemp Seeds & Microgreens is a versatile and balanced dish packed with healthy fats from the avocado, complete protein from the hemp seeds, and a vibrant array of vitamins and minerals from the microgreens. This anti-inflammatory recipe is quick to make, highly customizable, and perfect for anyone looking for a nutritious, plant-based meal. Add other toppings such as sliced tomatoes, radishes, or a poached egg to elevate the dish even further.

Golden Milk Smoothie Bowl

The *Golden Milk Smoothie Bowl* brings together the ancient healing power of turmeric, the star ingredient in golden milk, with a rich blend of fruits, nuts, and seeds for a delicious, nutrient-packed meal. This anti-inflammatory smoothie bowl is not only visually stunning with its bright golden color but also loaded with antioxidants, healthy fats, and plant-based protein. Turmeric, known for its powerful anti-inflammatory and antioxidant properties, is combined with warming spices like ginger and cinnamon to create a comforting, creamy smoothie base. It's perfect for breakfast or as a post-workout snack, and it provides long-lasting energy, digestive support, and overall well-being.

Preparation Time

- **Prep Time**: 10 minutes
- **Cook Time**: 0 minutes
- **Total Time**: 10 minutes

Ingredients

- 1 frozen banana
- 1/2 cup frozen mango chunks
- 1/2 cup unsweetened almond milk (or any plant-based milk)
- 1/2 teaspoon ground turmeric
- 1/4 teaspoon ground ginger (or a small piece of fresh ginger, peeled)
- 1/4 teaspoon ground cinnamon
- 1 tablespoon chia seeds

- 1 tablespoon almond butter (or any nut butter of choice)
- 1 teaspoon maple syrup (optional, for sweetness)
- 1/2 teaspoon vanilla extract (optional)

Toppings:

- Fresh fruit (such as berries, kiwi, or banana slices)
- Chia seeds or hemp seeds
- Granola or crushed nuts (almonds, walnuts, etc.)
- Coconut flakes
- A drizzle of honey or almond butter (optional)

Procedure

1. **Prepare the Smoothie Base**: In a blender, combine the frozen banana, frozen mango chunks, and unsweetened almond milk. Blend until smooth and creamy. The frozen fruit will give the smoothie bowl a thick, ice cream-like texture.
2. **Add the Spices**: Once the fruit is blended, add the ground turmeric, ground ginger, and cinnamon to the mix. These spices give the smoothie its signature "golden milk" flavor and provide potent anti-inflammatory and antioxidant benefits.
3. **Incorporate the Nutrients**: Add the chia seeds and almond butter for added fiber, healthy fats, and protein. Chia seeds help thicken the smoothie, while almond butter adds richness and creaminess. Blend again until everything is well incorporated.
4. **Adjust the Sweetness**: Taste the smoothie base, and if you prefer a sweeter flavor, add the maple syrup and vanilla extract. Blend briefly to mix the flavors.
5. **Pour into a Bowl**: Once the smoothie is smooth and thick, pour it into a bowl. The texture should be thick enough to hold up the toppings without sinking, creating the perfect smoothie bowl consistency.
6. **Add the Toppings**: Top the smoothie bowl with your choice of fresh fruit, such as berries, kiwi, or banana slices. Sprinkle on some chia seeds or hemp seeds for extra protein and fiber. Add granola or crushed nuts for crunch, and garnish with coconut flakes for a tropical twist.

7. **Finish and Serve**: For an extra touch, drizzle some honey or almond butter over the top. Serve immediately and enjoy this vibrant, nutrient-packed meal that's both refreshing and energizing.

Nutritional Value (per serving)

- **Calories**: ~320
- **Protein**: 8g
- **Carbohydrates**: 40g
- **Fiber**: 10g
- **Fat**: 16g
  - **Saturated Fat**: 2g
- **Sugar**: 25g (from fruit)
- **Sodium**: 100mg
- **Vitamin A**: 15% of daily recommended intake
- **Vitamin C**: 60% of daily recommended intake
- **Calcium**: 20% of daily recommended intake
- **Iron**: 8% of daily recommended intake

The *Golden Milk Smoothie Bowl* combines the anti-inflammatory benefits of turmeric and ginger with the creamy texture of frozen fruits and the richness of almond butter. This smoothie bowl is not only packed with essential vitamins and minerals but also provides a healthy dose of fiber, protein, and omega-3s from the chia seeds. It's perfect for boosting your immune system, supporting digestion, and fighting inflammation, while still being a delicious and satisfying treat. Enjoy it as a vibrant, nutrient-dense meal any time of day!

Quinoa Porridge with Cinnamon and Berries is a hearty, nutritious, and anti-inflammatory breakfast option that is perfect for starting your day on the right foot. Quinoa, a complete plant-based protein, is naturally gluten-free and packed with essential amino acids, fiber, and minerals like magnesium and iron. By using quinoa as the base for this porridge, you're creating a more nutrient-dense alternative to traditional oats. The addition of cinnamon, known for its anti-inflammatory properties, not only enhances the flavor but also helps regulate blood sugar levels. Fresh berries, rich in antioxidants, add a sweet and tangy finish, while the warmth of the cinnamon makes this dish comforting and energizing.

Preparation Time

- **Prep Time**: 5 minutes
- **Cook Time**: 15 minutes
- **Total Time**: 20 minutes

Ingredients

- 1 cup quinoa, rinsed and drained
- 2 cups unsweetened almond milk (or any plant-based milk)
- 1/2 teaspoon ground cinnamon
- 1/4 teaspoon vanilla extract (optional)
- 1 tablespoon maple syrup or honey (optional, for sweetness)
- 1/2 cup mixed fresh berries (blueberries, raspberries, strawberries, etc.)
- 1 tablespoon chia seeds (optional, for extra fiber and omega-3s)
- 1 tablespoon almond butter (optional, for extra creaminess)
- A pinch of salt
- Additional almond milk for serving (optional)

Procedure

1. **Cook the Quinoa**: In a medium-sized saucepan, combine the rinsed quinoa, almond milk, and a pinch of salt. Bring the mixture to a boil over medium heat, then reduce the heat to

low. Cover the saucepan and let the quinoa simmer for about 12–15 minutes, or until most of the liquid is absorbed and the quinoa becomes soft and fluffy.

2. **Add the Cinnamon and Flavorings**: Once the quinoa is cooked, stir in the ground cinnamon and vanilla extract (if using). These add a warm, sweet flavor to the porridge while boosting its anti-inflammatory properties. If you prefer a sweeter porridge, drizzle in the maple syrup or honey at this point.

3. **Simmer for Creaminess**: If the porridge is too thick for your liking, add a little more almond milk and continue to simmer the mixture until it reaches your desired consistency. The quinoa will absorb more liquid as it cooks, creating a creamy and comforting porridge base.

4. **Incorporate the Chia Seeds**: For added fiber and omega-3s, stir in a tablespoon of chia seeds. Let the porridge sit for a minute or two to allow the chia seeds to absorb some of the liquid, which will further thicken the texture.

5. **Serve the Porridge**: Spoon the warm quinoa porridge into individual bowls.

6. **Add the Toppings**: Top the porridge with a generous serving of fresh mixed berries for a burst of color, flavor, and antioxidants. For extra creaminess and healthy fats, drizzle almond butter on top or swirl it into the porridge.

7. **Garnish and Serve**: Finish by adding an extra splash of almond milk if you like a looser consistency, and sprinkle with additional cinnamon if desired. Serve warm and enjoy the comforting, nutrient-dense goodness of this anti-inflammatory porridge.

Nutritional Value (per serving)

- **Calories**: ~320
- **Protein**: 10g
- **Carbohydrates**: 50g
- **Fiber**: 8g
- **Fat**: 9g
    - o **Saturated Fat**: 1g
- **Sodium**: 100mg
- **Sugar**: 8g
- **Potassium**: 300mg

- **Calcium**: 20% of daily recommended intake
- **Iron**: 15% of daily recommended intake

Quinoa Porridge with Cinnamon and Berries is a complete meal that's rich in protein, fiber, and antioxidants, making it an ideal breakfast for anyone following an anti-inflammatory diet. The quinoa provides a slow-releasing source of energy that keeps you full and satisfied throughout the morning, while the berries add a sweet yet nutrient-packed touch. Cinnamon helps balance blood sugar, and the optional chia seeds and almond butter enhance the dish with additional healthy fats and nutrients. This porridge is a great way to incorporate plant-based protein into your diet while also enjoying a flavorful, comforting meal.

Flaxseed Banana Pancakes

Flaxseed Banana Pancakes are a delicious, nutrient-rich, and anti-inflammatory breakfast option that combines the natural sweetness of bananas with the health benefits of flaxseeds. Flaxseeds are high in omega-3 fatty acids and lignans, both of which help fight inflammation and support heart health. Bananas provide a good source of potassium and natural sweetness, reducing the need for added sugar in this recipe. These pancakes are not only gluten-free but also high in fiber, making them a perfect option for a filling and wholesome breakfast that will keep you satisfied and energized throughout the morning. Soft, fluffy, and mildly sweet, these pancakes are great for both adults and children and can be topped with a variety of healthy ingredients like berries, nut butter, or a drizzle of maple syrup.

Preparation Time

- **Prep Time**: 10 minutes
- **Cook Time**: 15 minutes
- **Total Time**: 25 minutes

Ingredients

- 2 ripe bananas, mashed
- 2 eggs
- 1/2 cup ground flaxseeds
- 1/2 cup almond flour (or any gluten-free flour)
- 1/2 teaspoon baking powder
- 1 teaspoon vanilla extract
- 1/2 teaspoon ground cinnamon
- 1/4 cup unsweetened almond milk (or any plant-based milk)
- 1 tablespoon maple syrup or honey (optional, for added sweetness)
- Coconut oil or olive oil for cooking

Optional Toppings:

- Fresh berries (such as blueberries or strawberries)
- Sliced bananas
- Nut butter (like almond or peanut butter)
- Chopped nuts
- A drizzle of maple syrup or honey

Procedure

1. **Mash the Bananas**: In a large mixing bowl, mash the ripe bananas until smooth. The riper the bananas, the sweeter and more flavorful your pancakes will be.

2. **Add the Wet Ingredients**: Add the eggs, vanilla extract, and almond milk to the mashed bananas, whisking until well combined. This mixture serves as the base for the pancake batter and will help bind the ingredients together.

3. **Mix in the Dry Ingredients**: In a separate bowl, combine the ground flaxseeds, almond flour, baking powder, and ground cinnamon. Stir the dry ingredients into the wet banana mixture, mixing just until everything is well combined. The flaxseeds will absorb some of the liquid, helping to thicken the batter.

4. **Let the Batter Rest**: Allow the pancake batter to sit for 5 minutes. This gives the flaxseeds time to absorb more liquid and create a thicker consistency, making the pancakes fluffier when cooked.

5. **Cook the Pancakes**: Heat a non-stick skillet or griddle over medium heat and add a small amount of coconut oil or olive oil to the pan. Pour about 1/4 cup of the batter onto the skillet for each pancake. Cook the pancakes for 2-3 minutes on each side, or until they are golden brown and cooked through.

6. **Flip with Care**: Because these pancakes are gluten-free, they may be a bit more delicate than traditional pancakes, so flip them gently to avoid breaking. Once both sides are cooked, remove the pancakes from the skillet and place them on a plate.

7. **Serve and Top**: Serve the pancakes warm and top with your favorite healthy toppings. Fresh berries, sliced bananas, nut butter, and a drizzle of maple syrup or honey all work wonderfully with the natural flavors of the pancakes.

Nutritional Value (per serving)

- **Calories**: ~270
- **Protein**: 10g
- **Carbohydrates**: 30g
- **Fiber**: 8g
- **Fat**: 14g
  - **Saturated Fat**: 2g
- **Sugar**: 12g (from natural fruit)
- **Sodium**: 150mg
- **Potassium**: 450mg
- **Omega-3 Fatty Acids**: 3g (from flaxseeds)
- **Vitamin C**: 10% of daily recommended intake
- **Calcium**: 15% of daily recommended intake
- **Iron**: 8% of daily recommended intake

Flaxseed Banana Pancakes are packed with fiber, protein, and healthy fats, making them a satisfying and nutrient-dense breakfast. The flaxseeds in this recipe provide a boost of omega-3 fatty acids, which support heart health and reduce inflammation. Bananas add natural sweetness and potassium, which is great for muscle function and maintaining healthy blood pressure. These pancakes are gluten-free, making them suitable for those with gluten sensitivities, and they're a great way to start the day with sustained energy and balanced nutrition. Add a variety of toppings to customize the flavor and make this meal even more enjoyable.

Anti-Inflammatory Green Smoothie

The *Anti-Inflammatory Green Smoothie* is a powerhouse of nutrition, blending vibrant leafy greens, antioxidant-rich fruits, and inflammation-fighting ingredients into one delicious, refreshing drink. This smoothie is perfect for starting your day with a burst of nutrients, supporting your immune system, and reducing inflammation in the body. The base of the smoothie typically includes spinach or kale, which are loaded with vitamins A, C, and K, as well as magnesium and antioxidants. Ginger and turmeric, both renowned for their anti-inflammatory properties, bring warmth and spice to the mix. Paired with hydrating coconut water and the natural sweetness of fruits like pineapple and banana, this smoothie balances health with flavor.

Preparation Time

- **Prep Time**: 5 minutes
- **Cook Time**: 0 minutes
- **Total Time**: 5 minutes

Ingredients

- 1 cup fresh spinach (or kale)
- 1/2 cup frozen pineapple chunks
- 1/2 banana (fresh or frozen)
- 1/2 teaspoon ground turmeric
- 1/2 teaspoon freshly grated ginger (or 1/4 teaspoon ground ginger)
- 1 tablespoon ground flaxseeds or chia seeds
- 1 cup coconut water (or unsweetened almond milk)
- 1/2 teaspoon cinnamon (optional, for flavor and added anti-inflammatory benefit)
- 1 teaspoon honey or maple syrup (optional, for sweetness)

- Ice cubes (optional, for a colder smoothie)

Procedure

1. **Prepare the Ingredients**: Start by washing and prepping your fresh ingredients. If you're using fresh ginger, peel and grate a small piece. Ensure the spinach or kale is thoroughly rinsed and ready to blend.

2. **Add the Greens**: In a blender, add the fresh spinach or kale as the base. Leafy greens are packed with antioxidants, vitamins, and minerals that support overall health and fight inflammation.

3. **Incorporate the Fruit**: Add the frozen pineapple chunks and banana to the blender. These fruits bring natural sweetness to balance out the greens and are loaded with vitamin C and potassium, which further support anti-inflammatory effects.

4. **Spice It Up with Turmeric and Ginger**: Add the ground turmeric and freshly grated ginger to the mix. These two powerful anti-inflammatory ingredients help reduce oxidative stress and inflammation in the body. Turmeric contains curcumin, which has been shown to reduce markers of inflammation, while ginger soothes the digestive system.

5. **Boost with Seeds**: Add the ground flaxseeds or chia seeds, which provide omega-3 fatty acids, fiber, and protein. These help reduce inflammation, support heart health, and keep you feeling full longer.

6. **Blend with Liquid**: Pour in the coconut water (or almond milk) to help blend everything together. Coconut water is hydrating and rich in potassium, making it an excellent base for this smoothie. Blend until smooth. If you prefer a colder smoothie, add a few ice cubes before blending.

7. **Taste and Adjust**: After blending, taste the smoothie. If you prefer it sweeter, add a teaspoon of honey or maple syrup. For extra flavor, you can also sprinkle in some cinnamon, which has additional anti-inflammatory properties. Blend again briefly to incorporate any additional ingredients, then serve immediately.

Nutritional Value (per serving)

- **Calories**: ~210
- **Protein**: 4g
- **Carbohydrates**: 38g
- **Fiber**: 7g
- **Fat**: 5g
- **Saturated Fat**: 0.5g
- **Sugar**: 16g (from fruit)
- **Sodium**: 80mg
- **Potassium**: 600mg
- **Vitamin A**: 70% of daily recommended intake
- **Vitamin C**: 110% of daily recommended intake
- **Calcium**: 8% of daily recommended intake
- **Iron**: 10% of daily recommended intake
- **Omega-3 Fatty Acids**: 2.5g (from flaxseeds)

The *Anti-Inflammatory Green Smoothie* is a nutrient-dense drink that can help reduce inflammation, support digestion, and provide a quick energy boost. The leafy greens are rich in fiber and antioxidants, while turmeric and ginger offer powerful anti-inflammatory compounds that promote healing and reduce joint pain. Pineapple and banana not only add natural sweetness but also supply essential vitamins and minerals that support heart health and immune function. This smoothie is also a great source of omega-3s from the flaxseeds or chia seeds, making it a well-rounded and delicious way to start your day or recover post-workout.

Chapter 2

Energizing Snacks & Small Bites

Turmeric Roasted Chickpeas

Turmeric Roasted Chickpeas are a flavorful, crunchy, and nutrient-packed snack or topping that is perfect for boosting your intake of anti-inflammatory foods. Chickpeas, also known as garbanzo beans, are rich in plant-based protein, fiber, and essential vitamins and minerals. When roasted, they become crispy on the outside while maintaining a chewy center, making them an excellent alternative to less healthy snacks like chips. Turmeric, the star spice in this recipe, contains curcumin, a powerful anti-inflammatory compound that has been shown to reduce inflammation and oxidative stress in the body. Combined with olive oil and other spices like paprika and garlic powder, this simple recipe transforms chickpeas into a delicious and health-supportive treat. These roasted chickpeas are great for snacking, adding crunch to salads, or using as a topping for soups or grain bowls.

Preparation Time

- **Prep Time**: 5 minutes
- **Cook Time**: 30 minutes
- **Total Time**: 35 minutes

Ingredients

- 1 can (15 ounces) chickpeas, drained and rinsed
- 1 tablespoon olive oil
- 1 teaspoon ground turmeric
- 1/2 teaspoon ground cumin
- 1/2 teaspoon smoked paprika (or regular paprika)
- 1/2 teaspoon garlic powder
- 1/4 teaspoon ground black pepper
- Salt, to taste

Procedure

1. **Prepare the Chickpeas**: Start by draining and rinsing the canned chickpeas under cold water. Pat them dry with a clean kitchen towel or paper towels. The drier the chickpeas, the crispier they will become when roasted. Removing excess moisture is key to achieving the desired crunch.

2. **Preheat the Oven**: Preheat your oven to 400°F (200°C). Line a baking sheet with parchment paper or lightly grease it with olive oil to prevent the chickpeas from sticking.

3. **Season the Chickpeas**: In a medium bowl, toss the dried chickpeas with olive oil to coat them evenly. Then add the ground turmeric, cumin, smoked paprika, garlic powder, black pepper, and a pinch of salt. Stir until the chickpeas are well coated with the spices. Turmeric brings its signature golden color and anti-inflammatory benefits, while cumin and paprika add warmth and depth of flavor.

4. **Spread on Baking Sheet**: Spread the seasoned chickpeas in an even layer on the prepared baking sheet. Make sure they are not overlapping, as this will help them roast evenly and become crispier.

5. **Roast the Chickpeas**: Place the baking sheet in the preheated oven and roast for 25–30 minutes, shaking the pan or stirring the chickpeas halfway through to ensure they roast evenly. The chickpeas should become golden and crispy on the outside.

6. **Check for Doneness**: After about 30 minutes, check the chickpeas for doneness. They should be crisp and slightly browned. If they are not crispy enough, you can leave them in the oven for an additional 5–10 minutes, but be careful not to burn them.

7. **Cool and Serve**: Once the chickpeas are fully roasted, remove them from the oven and let them cool for a few minutes. They will continue to crisp up as they cool. Serve immediately as a snack or store in an airtight container for up to 3–4 days. Enjoy them on their own, or use them to add crunch to salads, soups, or grain bowls.

Nutritional Value (per 1/2 cup serving)

- **Calories**: ~140
- **Protein**: 6g
- **Carbohydrates**: 20g

- **Fiber**: 6g
- **Fat**: 5g
- **Saturated Fat**: 0.5g
- **Sugar**: 1g
- **Sodium**: 200mg (varies depending on added salt)
- **Potassium**: 220mg
- **Iron**: 10% of daily recommended intake
- **Calcium**: 4% of daily recommended intake
- **Vitamin C**: 2% of daily recommended intake

Turmeric Roasted Chickpeas are a healthy, flavorful, and satisfying snack that offers a great balance of protein and fiber, making them filling and perfect for curbing cravings. The fiber in chickpeas supports digestive health, while the protein makes this snack ideal for boosting energy. Turmeric, with its anti-inflammatory curcumin content, helps reduce inflammation in the body, and the added spices like cumin and paprika enhance both the flavor and the health benefits. These roasted chickpeas are versatile and can be enjoyed on their own or as a crunchy addition to a variety of dishes, making them a tasty and functional part of any anti-inflammatory diet.

Avocado-Stuffed Bell Peppers are a vibrant, nutrient-dense, and anti-inflammatory dish that combines the healthy fats of avocado with the refreshing crunch of bell peppers. Bell peppers are rich in vitamins A and C, providing antioxidants that support immune health and reduce inflammation. Avocados offer heart-healthy monounsaturated fats and fiber, helping to regulate cholesterol levels and keep you feeling full. This recipe can be served as a light lunch, a side dish, or even a snack, and is packed with a variety of flavors and textures. The creaminess of the avocado is perfectly balanced by the crispness of the raw bell peppers, while additional ingredients like lime juice, cilantro, and spices give this dish a zesty and fresh flavor. This recipe is naturally gluten-free, vegan, and can be easily customized by adding protein or other toppings.

Preparation Time

- **Prep Time**: 10 minutes
- **Cook Time**: 0 minutes
- **Total Time**: 10 minutes

Ingredients

- 4 medium bell peppers (red, yellow, or orange), halved and seeds removed
- 2 large ripe avocados
- 1 small red onion, finely diced
- 1 small tomato, diced
- 1/4 cup fresh cilantro, chopped
- Juice of 1 lime
- 1/2 teaspoon ground cumin
- 1/2 teaspoon garlic powder
- Salt and pepper, to taste
- Optional toppings: jalapeño slices, diced cucumber, crumbled feta cheese (optional), or a sprinkle of chili flakes for extra heat

Procedure

1. **Prepare the Bell Peppers**: Begin by washing the bell peppers thoroughly. Slice them in half lengthwise and remove the seeds and inner membranes. Set the bell pepper halves aside, which will serve as the vessels for the avocado filling. Bell peppers are rich in antioxidants, especially vitamin C, making them a perfect base for this dish.

2. **Mash the Avocados**: In a medium mixing bowl, scoop out the flesh of the ripe avocados. Mash them with a fork until smooth but slightly chunky, retaining some texture. Avocados are the heart of this dish, providing healthy fats and a creamy texture that complements the crisp bell peppers.

3. **Add the Vegetables**: To the mashed avocado, add the diced red onion, tomato, and cilantro. The red onion adds a mild sharpness, while the tomatoes offer a juicy, slightly sweet contrast. Cilantro brings freshness to the mix and enhances the overall flavor profile.

4. **Season with Spices**: Add the ground cumin, garlic powder, lime juice, and a pinch of salt and pepper to the avocado mixture. These spices not only enhance the taste but also add anti-inflammatory benefits. Lime juice brightens the flavors and prevents the avocado from browning. Stir until everything is well combined.

5. **Stuff the Bell Peppers**: Using a spoon, evenly divide the avocado mixture and stuff each bell pepper half. The creamy avocado filling pairs perfectly with the crispness of the raw bell peppers, creating a delicious contrast of textures.

6. **Garnish and Customize**: Add optional toppings like jalapeño slices for heat, crumbled feta cheese for a salty kick, or diced cucumber for added crunch. You can also sprinkle chili flakes for a touch of spice if desired. This step allows you to personalize the dish according to your taste preferences.

7. **Serve and Enjoy**: Serve the avocado-stuffed bell peppers immediately. These stuffed peppers can be enjoyed as a refreshing snack, a light meal, or a colorful appetizer. They're best eaten fresh but can also be stored in the refrigerator for up to a day.

Nutritional Value (per serving, 2 stuffed pepper halves)

- **Calories**: ~200
- **Protein**: 3g
- **Carbohydrates**: 15g
- **Fiber**: 8g
- **Fat**: 15g
- **Saturated Fat**: 2g
- **Sugar**: 5g (from bell peppers)
- **Sodium**: 150mg
- **Potassium**: 650mg
- **Vitamin A**: 100% of daily recommended intake
- **Vitamin C**: 250% of daily recommended intake
- **Calcium**: 5% of daily recommended intake
- **Iron**: 6% of daily recommended intake

Avocado-Stuffed Bell Peppers are a fantastic low-carb, nutrient-rich dish that provides a wide range of health benefits. The avocado is packed with heart-healthy fats and fiber, which support healthy digestion and reduce inflammation. Bell peppers are an excellent source of antioxidants, particularly vitamin C, which supports the immune system and skin health. This recipe is also high in fiber, making it satisfying and beneficial for gut health. Whether served as a light meal or snack, these stuffed peppers are a refreshing, flavorful, and nutritious addition to an anti-inflammatory diet.

Cucumber Hummus Bites are a refreshing, light, and nutritious snack perfect for any time of day. Combining the cool, crisp texture of cucumber with the creamy, protein-rich hummus, this snack provides a burst of flavor and a variety of nutrients. Cucumbers are low in calories but high in hydration, offering a cooling crunch that's ideal for pairing with savory dips like hummus. Hummus, made from chickpeas, tahini, olive oil, and lemon juice, is not only delicious but also loaded with plant-based protein, healthy fats, and fiber. These bites are quick to assemble, making them a great appetizer for parties, an afternoon snack, or even part of a light meal. The dish is naturally vegan, gluten-free, and customizable with various toppings such as cherry tomatoes, olives, or herbs to suit different tastes. It's a wonderful addition to an anti-inflammatory diet, thanks to the nutrient-dense ingredients that support heart and digestive health.

Preparation Time

- **Prep Time**: 10 minutes
- **Cook Time**: 0 minutes
- **Total Time**: 10 minutes

Ingredients

- 1 large cucumber
- 1/2 cup hummus (store-bought or homemade)
- 1 tablespoon olive oil (optional, for drizzling)
- 1 teaspoon paprika or smoked paprika (optional, for garnish)
- 1 tablespoon fresh parsley or cilantro, chopped (for garnish)
- 6–8 cherry tomatoes, halved (optional topping)
- 1 tablespoon sesame seeds or hemp seeds (optional, for garnish)
- Salt and pepper, to taste

Procedure

1. **Prepare the Cucumber**: Wash the cucumber thoroughly and cut it into thick, round slices, about 1/2-inch each. These slices will serve as the base for the hummus bites, providing a crisp and hydrating foundation. You can peel the cucumber or leave the skin on for added fiber and nutrients.

2. **Prepare the Hummus**: If using store-bought hummus, give it a quick stir. If you're making homemade hummus, blend chickpeas, tahini, lemon juice, olive oil, garlic, and salt in a food processor until smooth. Hummus offers a creamy, nutrient-dense spread packed with protein, fiber, and healthy fats.

3. **Assemble the Bites**: Place about 1 teaspoon of hummus on each cucumber slice. Spread it out evenly over the top. You can use more or less hummus, depending on your preference. The combination of cucumber and hummus provides a contrast between the cool, refreshing base and the creamy topping.

4. **Add Toppings**: For added flavor and texture, garnish the hummus bites with a sprinkle of paprika or smoked paprika. This adds a mild, spicy kick and vibrant color. Drizzle a little olive oil on top if desired for extra richness and healthy fats.

5. **Garnish with Fresh Herbs**: Sprinkle freshly chopped parsley or cilantro over the hummus bites. Fresh herbs not only enhance the flavor but also add a bright, fresh note and additional antioxidants to this already nutrient-rich snack.

6. **Customize with Additional Toppings**: Add optional toppings like halved cherry tomatoes for a pop of color and sweetness, or sprinkle sesame seeds or hemp seeds for a bit of crunch and extra protein. These toppings also provide additional healthy fats and micronutrients.

7. **Serve and Enjoy**: Arrange the cucumber hummus bites on a serving plate and sprinkle a pinch of salt and pepper over the top to taste. Serve immediately to retain the freshness of the cucumber. These bites are a great snack or appetizer and can be refrigerated for a few hours if needed.

Nutritional Value (per 6 cucumber hummus bites)

- **Calories**: ~80
- **Protein**: 3g
- **Carbohydrates**: 8g
- **Fiber**: 3g
- **Fat**: 4g
- **Saturated Fat**: 0.5g
- **Sugar**: 2g
- **Sodium**: 150mg
- **Potassium**: 250mg
- **Vitamin A**: 6% of daily recommended intake
- **Vitamin C**: 12% of daily recommended intake
- **Calcium**: 4% of daily recommended intake
- **Iron**: 6% of daily recommended intake

Cucumber Hummus Bites are a perfect snack or appetizer for those looking for a healthy, low-calorie option packed with nutrients. The cucumbers provide hydration and a crisp, refreshing base that complements the creamy, protein-rich hummus. Hummus, made from chickpeas, offers plant-based protein and fiber that help keep you full while supporting digestive health. With additional anti-inflammatory benefits from the olive oil, paprika, and herbs, this dish is both nutritious and delicious. Customizable with various toppings, these bites are not only visually appealing but also incredibly versatile, making them an ideal part of an anti-inflammatory diet.

Walnut & Berry Energy Bites are a delicious and nutritious snack packed with energy-boosting ingredients. These no-bake bites combine the richness of walnuts with the natural sweetness of dried berries, making them an ideal snack for any time of the day. Walnuts are an excellent source of omega-3 fatty acids, which are known for their anti-inflammatory properties, as well as protein and fiber. Dried berries, such as cranberries, blueberries, or goji berries, provide antioxidants and vitamins that support overall health. These energy bites are quick and easy to prepare, making them perfect for busy lifestyles. They are naturally sweetened with honey or maple syrup, giving them a delightful flavor without the need for refined sugars. Whether you need a pre-workout boost, a mid-afternoon snack, or a healthy treat, these energy bites offer a wholesome solution.

Preparation Time

- **Prep Time**: 15 minutes
- **Cook Time**: 0 minutes
- **Total Time**: 15 minutes

Ingredients

- 1 cup walnuts
- 1 cup rolled oats
- 1/2 cup dried mixed berries (e.g., cranberries, blueberries, or goji berries)
- 1/4 cup honey or maple syrup (for a vegan option)
- 1/2 teaspoon vanilla extract
- 1/4 teaspoon ground cinnamon
- Pinch of salt
- Optional: 1/4 cup unsweetened shredded coconut or chia seeds for rolling

Procedure

1. **Prepare the Walnuts**: Start by placing the walnuts in a food processor. Pulse them until they are finely chopped but not ground into a powder. The walnuts provide healthy fats and protein, contributing to the energy-boosting properties of these bites.

2. **Combine Ingredients**: In a large mixing bowl, combine the chopped walnuts, rolled oats, dried mixed berries, honey or maple syrup, vanilla extract, ground cinnamon, and a pinch of salt. This mixture will create a sticky, flavorful base for the energy bites.

3. **Mix Thoroughly**: Using a spatula or your hands, mix the ingredients until everything is well combined. Ensure the oats and walnuts are evenly distributed, and the dried berries are fully incorporated. The sticky sweetener will help bind the ingredients together.

4. **Form the Bites**: With clean hands, scoop out about 1 tablespoon of the mixture and roll it into a ball. Repeat this process until all the mixture is used. The size of the bites can be adjusted to your preference, but keeping them around 1-inch in diameter makes them easy to eat.

5. **Coat the Bites (Optional)**: If desired, roll the energy bites in shredded coconut or chia seeds for an extra layer of texture and nutrition. This step adds healthy fats and additional fiber, enhancing the nutritional profile of the bites.

6. **Chill the Bites**: Place the energy bites on a plate or a baking sheet lined with parchment paper. Refrigerate them for about 30 minutes to help them firm up. Chilling will enhance their texture, making them easier to store and eat later.

7. **Store and Enjoy**: After chilling, transfer the energy bites to an airtight container. They can be stored in the refrigerator for up to a week or frozen for longer shelf life. Enjoy these bites as a quick snack on the go or as a healthy treat anytime you need an energy boost.

Nutritional Value (per energy bite, approximately 1-inch in diameter)

- **Calories**: ~100
- **Protein**: 3g
- **Carbohydrates**: 12g
- **Fiber**: 2g
- **Fat**: 5g
- **Saturated Fat**: 0.5g
- **Sugar**: 4g (from honey/maple syrup and dried berries)
- **Sodium**: 0mg
- **Potassium**: 100mg
- **Vitamin E**: 5% of daily recommended intake

- **Iron**: 4% of daily recommended intake
- **Calcium**: 2% of daily recommended intake

Walnut & Berry Energy Bites are an excellent choice for anyone seeking a wholesome snack that is both nutritious and satisfying. With the combination of walnuts and oats, these bites offer a balanced source of protein and healthy fats, making them great for energy and satiety. Dried berries provide a natural sweetness and a burst of antioxidants, enhancing the health benefits of the snack. Whether you're preparing for a workout or need a quick pick-me-up during the day, these energy bites are easy to make and provide a nutritious option without refined sugars. Their versatility allows for various customizations, so feel free to swap in your favorite nuts or dried fruits. With their delightful flavor and satisfying texture, these energy bites are sure to become a favorite in your kitchen.

Crispy Kale Chips with Nutritional Yeast

Crispy Kale Chips with Nutritional Yeast are a healthy, crunchy snack that's perfect for satisfying cravings without the guilt. Kale is one of the most nutrient-dense vegetables available, packed with vitamins A, C, and K, along with antioxidants that promote overall health. Nutritional yeast adds a cheesy, umami flavor to the kale chips while providing a boost of B vitamins, including B12, which is particularly beneficial for those following a vegan diet. This recipe is quick and simple, allowing you to transform fresh kale into a flavorful snack in no time. Whether enjoyed on their own, sprinkled over salads, or used as a topping for soups, these kale chips offer a delicious way to incorporate more greens into your diet. They're naturally low in calories and high in fiber, making them an ideal choice for anyone looking to maintain a healthy lifestyle.

Preparation Time

- **Prep Time**: 10 minutes
- **Cook Time**: 15 minutes
- **Total Time**: 25 minutes

Ingredients

- 1 bunch of kale (approximately 8-10 ounces)
- 1 tablespoon olive oil
- 2-3 tablespoons nutritional yeast
- 1/2 teaspoon garlic powder
- 1/2 teaspoon onion powder
- 1/4 teaspoon smoked paprika (optional, for a smoky flavor)
- Salt and pepper, to taste

Procedure

1. **Preheat the Oven**: Begin by preheating your oven to 350°F (175°C). A hot oven is essential for achieving the perfect crispiness without burning the kale chips.

2. **Prepare the Kale**: Rinse the kale thoroughly under cool water to remove any dirt or debris. Pat the leaves dry with a clean kitchen towel or use a salad spinner to remove excess moisture. Drying the kale well is crucial for ensuring that the chips become crispy during baking.

3. **Remove the Stems**: Tear the kale leaves from the thick stems and into bite-sized pieces. Discard the stems, as they can be tough and chewy. This step ensures that you only use the tender leaves, which will become delightfully crispy in the oven.

4. **Massage with Oil**: In a large mixing bowl, combine the kale pieces with olive oil. Use your hands to massage the oil into the leaves, ensuring that each piece is evenly coated. This helps the kale to bake evenly and enhances the flavor of the final product.

5. **Season the Kale**: Sprinkle the nutritional yeast, garlic powder, onion powder, smoked paprika (if using), salt, and pepper over the kale. Toss everything together until the kale is well coated with the seasonings. Nutritional yeast adds a cheesy flavor that pairs wonderfully with the kale.

6. **Spread on a Baking Sheet**: Arrange the seasoned kale in a single layer on a baking sheet lined with parchment paper. Avoid overcrowding the pan, as this will prevent the kale from crisping up. If you have too much kale, consider using two baking sheets or baking in batches.

7. **Bake and Serve**: Place the baking sheet in the preheated oven and bake for 10-15 minutes, or until the kale chips are crispy and lightly browned. Keep an eye on them to prevent burning, as they can quickly go from perfect to overdone. Once baked, remove them from the oven and let them cool for a few minutes before serving. Enjoy these kale chips on their own or as a tasty topping for salads and soups!

Nutritional Value (per serving, approximately 1 ounce or 28g)

- **Calories**: ~100
- **Protein**: 4g
- **Carbohydrates**: 6g
- **Fiber**: 2g
- **Fat**: 7g
- **Saturated Fat**: 1g
- **Sugar**: 1g
- **Sodium**: 200mg (depending on added salt)
- **Potassium**: 300mg
- **Vitamin A**: 150% of daily recommended intake
- **Vitamin C**: 10% of daily recommended intake
- **Calcium**: 4% of daily recommended intake
- **Iron**: 6% of daily recommended intake

Crispy Kale Chips with Nutritional Yeast are a nutritious and flavorful snack that is incredibly easy to prepare. The kale provides a wealth of vitamins and minerals, while the nutritional yeast gives a satisfying cheesy flavor without the dairy. This snack is perfect for those following a vegan or plant-based diet and is low in calories, making it suitable for weight management. The addition of garlic and onion powder enhances the overall taste, providing a savory depth that complements the natural flavor of the kale. These chips are versatile and can be enjoyed on their own, crumbled over salads, or as a crunchy topping for soups. By making these kale chips at home, you can enjoy a healthy alternative to traditional chips, satisfying your cravings while supporting your wellness journey.

The *Golden Glow Smoothie* is a vibrant and refreshing drink that combines the tropical sweetness of mango with the warm, spicy flavors of ginger and turmeric. This smoothie is not only delicious but also packed with nutrients that promote overall health and wellness. Mango is rich in vitamins A and C, providing essential antioxidants that support immune function and skin health. Ginger adds a spicy kick and is known for its anti-inflammatory properties, making it an excellent choice for digestive health. Turmeric, often hailed as a superfood, contains curcumin, which has powerful anti-inflammatory and antioxidant benefits. Together, these ingredients create a smoothie that is not only visually appealing but also a powerhouse of nutrition. Enjoy it as a breakfast option, a post-workout refreshment, or a delightful afternoon pick-me-up.

Preparation Time

- **Prep Time**: 10 minutes
- **Cook Time**: 0 minutes
- **Total Time**: 10 minutes

Ingredients

- 1 ripe mango, peeled and diced (fresh or frozen)
- 1/2 banana (fresh or frozen)
- 1 teaspoon fresh ginger, grated (or 1/4 teaspoon ground ginger)
- 1/2 teaspoon ground turmeric (or 1 teaspoon fresh turmeric, grated)
- 1 cup unsweetened almond milk (or any milk of choice)
- 1 tablespoon honey or maple syrup (optional, for sweetness)
- 1/2 cup ice cubes (optional, for a thicker texture)
- Pinch of black pepper (to enhance turmeric absorption)
- Optional toppings: chia seeds, coconut flakes, or sliced almonds

Procedure

1. **Prepare the Ingredients**: Gather all the ingredients and, if using fresh produce, peel and dice the mango and banana. Grate the fresh ginger and turmeric, or measure out the ground spices. This preparation step ensures that everything is ready to blend smoothly.

2. **Blend the Base**: In a high-speed blender, combine the diced mango, banana, grated ginger, and turmeric. These ingredients create a flavorful and nutrient-dense base for the smoothie.

3. **Add the Liquid**: Pour in the almond milk (or your preferred milk) to help the blending process. The liquid component is essential for achieving the desired creamy consistency of the smoothie.

4. **Sweeten the Smoothie**: If you prefer a sweeter smoothie, add honey or maple syrup to taste. This step is optional, as the natural sweetness of the mango and banana may be sufficient.

5. **Incorporate Ice (if desired)**: For a thicker, frostier texture, add ice cubes to the blender. This will make the smoothie refreshing, especially on warm days.

6. **Blend Until Smooth**: Secure the lid on the blender and blend on high speed until all the ingredients are fully combined and the mixture is smooth and creamy. Stop to scrape down the sides if necessary to ensure everything is well incorporated.

7. **Serve and Enjoy**: Pour the smoothie into a glass, and if desired, sprinkle with optional toppings such as chia seeds, coconut flakes, or sliced almonds for added texture and nutrition. Enjoy immediately for the best flavor and freshness!

Nutritional Value (per serving, approximately 1 cup)

- **Calories**: ~210
- **Protein**: 3g
- **Carbohydrates**: 43g
- **Fiber**: 5g
- **Fat**: 3g
- **Saturated Fat**: 0.5g
- **Sugar**: 24g
- **Sodium**: 50mg

- **Potassium**: 550mg
- **Vitamin A**: 20% of daily recommended intake
- **Vitamin C**: 70% of daily recommended intake
- **Calcium**: 6% of daily recommended intake
- **Iron**: 4% of daily recommended intake

The *Golden Glow Smoothie* is a delightful way to nourish your body while enjoying the vibrant flavors of mango, ginger, and turmeric. This smoothie not only tastes fantastic but also provides a host of health benefits, including anti-inflammatory properties and essential vitamins. The combination of mango and banana creates a naturally sweet and creamy base, while ginger adds a zesty kick that invigorates your palate. Turmeric, known for its bright golden hue, enhances the drink's visual appeal and brings powerful health benefits. With optional toppings, you can easily customize this smoothie to suit your taste preferences. Whether you're looking for a healthy breakfast, a post-workout boost, or a refreshing afternoon snack, this smoothie is sure to become a staple in your diet. Enjoy the golden goodness and the energy it brings!

Spiced Carrot and Almond Muffins

Spiced Carrot and Almond Muffins are a delightful blend of flavors and textures that make for a perfect breakfast or snack option. These muffins are packed with the natural sweetness of grated carrots, which not only add moisture but also provide essential vitamins and antioxidants. Almonds introduce a satisfying crunch while contributing healthy fats and protein, making these muffins a well-rounded treat. The warm spices, including cinnamon and nutmeg, elevate the flavor profile, creating a comforting and aromatic experience. Perfectly moist and tender, these muffins are easy to prepare and can be made in batches for quick grab-and-go options. Whether enjoyed fresh out of the oven or stored for later, these muffins are sure to please both adults and children alike. They are also versatile, allowing for the addition of optional ingredients like raisins or coconut to suit your taste preferences.

Preparation Time

- **Prep Time**: 15 minutes
- **Cook Time**: 20-25 minutes
- **Total Time**: 35-40 minutes

Ingredients

- 1 cup whole wheat flour
- 1/2 cup almond flour
- 1 teaspoon baking powder
- 1/2 teaspoon baking soda
- 1 teaspoon ground cinnamon
- 1/2 teaspoon ground nutmeg
- 1/4 teaspoon salt
- 1/2 cup honey or maple syrup (for a vegan option)
- 2 large eggs (or flax eggs for a vegan option)
- 1/3 cup unsweetened applesauce
- 1 teaspoon vanilla extract
- 1 cup grated carrots (about 2 medium carrots)
- 1/2 cup chopped almonds (or walnuts, if preferred)
- Optional: 1/4 cup raisins or dried cranberries

Procedure

1. **Preheat the Oven**: Begin by preheating your oven to 350°F (175°C). This step is crucial to ensure the muffins bake evenly and rise properly.
2. **Prepare Muffin Tin**: Grease a muffin tin or line it with paper liners to prevent sticking. This will make for easy removal and cleanup after baking.
3. **Mix Dry Ingredients**: In a large mixing bowl, combine the whole wheat flour, almond flour, baking powder, baking soda, cinnamon, nutmeg, and salt. Whisk the dry ingredients together to ensure they are well mixed and to aerate the flour.

4. **Combine Wet Ingredients**: In a separate bowl, whisk together the honey or maple syrup, eggs (or flax eggs), applesauce, and vanilla extract until smooth. This mixture will add moisture and sweetness to the muffins.

5. **Combine Mixtures**: Pour the wet ingredients into the bowl with the dry ingredients. Gently fold the two mixtures together until just combined, being careful not to overmix, as this can result in dense muffins.

6. **Add Carrots and Nuts**: Fold in the grated carrots and chopped almonds (and raisins, if using) until evenly distributed throughout the batter. The carrots will add moisture, while the almonds provide a nice crunch and flavor.

7. **Bake and Cool**: Divide the batter evenly among the muffin cups, filling each about 2/3 full. Bake in the preheated oven for 20-25 minutes, or until a toothpick inserted into the center comes out clean. Allow the muffins to cool in the tin for a few minutes before transferring them to a wire rack to cool completely. Enjoy them warm or store them in an airtight container for later!

Nutritional Value (per muffin, approximately 1 muffin)

- **Calories**: ~180
- **Protein**: 4g
- **Carbohydrates**: 25g
- **Fiber**: 3g
- **Fat**: 8g
- **Saturated Fat**: 0.5g
- **Sugar**: 8g (depending on added sweetener)
- **Sodium**: 180mg
- **Potassium**: 150mg
- **Vitamin A**: 45% of daily recommended intake
- **Calcium**: 4% of daily recommended intake
- **Iron**: 6% of daily recommended intake

Spiced Carrot and Almond Muffins are a delicious way to enjoy wholesome ingredients while satisfying your sweet tooth. These muffins are rich in vitamins, minerals, and healthy fats, making them a nourishing option for any time of day. The use of whole wheat and almond flour enhances the nutritional profile, providing fiber and protein that will keep you fuller for longer. The warm spices create a comforting aroma and flavor, making these muffins feel like a treat while still being nutritious. They are perfect for breakfast on the go, a midday snack, or even a light dessert. With their delightful taste and health benefits, these muffins are sure to become a favorite in your recipe collection. Customize them with your favorite mix-ins, and enjoy the goodness of carrots and almonds in every bite!

Coconut and Matcha Protein Bars

Coconut and Matcha Protein Bars are a nutritious and energizing snack that combines the tropical flavor of coconut with the earthy notes of matcha green tea. These bars are packed with protein, making them an ideal post-workout treat or a satisfying snack to fuel your day. Matcha is known for its rich antioxidant content and metabolism-boosting properties, while coconut adds healthy fats and a delightful chewiness. The combination of these ingredients creates a deliciously sweet yet health-conscious snack that is easy to prepare at home. Whether you're on the go or need a quick pick-me-up, these protein bars provide a perfect balance of nutrients to keep you energized. Plus, they are naturally sweetened, making them a healthier alternative to store-bought protein bars filled with additives and preservatives. Enjoy them as a part of your meal prep for the week, and indulge in their guilt-free goodness!

Preparation Time

- **Prep Time**: 15 minutes
- **Cook Time**: 10 minutes
- **Total Time**: 25 minutes

Ingredients

- 1 cup rolled oats
- 1/2 cup unsweetened shredded coconut
- 1/2 cup almond or peanut butter
- 1/4 cup honey or maple syrup (for a vegan option)
- 2 tablespoons matcha powder
- 1/4 cup protein powder (vanilla or unflavored)
- 1/4 teaspoon salt
- Optional: 1/4 cup dark chocolate chips or chopped nuts for added texture

Procedure

1. **Prepare the Baking Dish**: Start by lining an 8x8-inch baking dish with parchment paper, allowing some overhang for easy removal later. This will prevent the protein bars from sticking to the dish and make cutting them easier.

2. **Mix Dry Ingredients**: In a large mixing bowl, combine the rolled oats, shredded coconut, matcha powder, protein powder, and salt. Whisk the dry ingredients together until well mixed, ensuring the matcha is evenly distributed throughout the mixture.

3. **Combine Wet Ingredients**: In a separate bowl, mix together the almond or peanut butter and honey (or maple syrup) until smooth and well combined. This mixture will serve as the binding agent for the bars.

4. **Combine Mixtures**: Pour the wet mixture into the bowl with the dry ingredients. Stir well until all ingredients are thoroughly combined and the oats and coconut are evenly coated. If using, fold in the chocolate chips or nuts at this stage for added flavor and texture.

5. **Press into the Dish**: Transfer the mixture into the prepared baking dish. Use a spatula or your hands to press the mixture firmly and evenly into the dish. Pressing down helps the bars hold their shape after being cut.

6. **Bake**: Preheat your oven to 350°F (175°C). Bake the bars in the oven for 10 minutes, just enough to firm them up without drying them out.

7. **Cool and Cut**: Once baked, remove the dish from the oven and allow the bars to cool completely in the dish. Once cool, use the parchment paper overhang to lift the bars out and place them on a cutting board. Cut into squares or rectangles, and store them in an airtight container in the refrigerator for up to a week. Enjoy your homemade protein bars as a convenient snack or energy boost throughout the week!

Nutritional Value (per bar, approximately 1 bar from 12 servings)

- **Calories**: ~150
- **Protein**: 5g
- **Carbohydrates**: 20g
- **Fiber**: 3g
- **Fat**: 7g
- **Saturated Fat**: 3g
- **Sugar**: 6g (depending on added sweetener)
- **Sodium**: 50mg
- **Potassium**: 150mg
- **Calcium**: 4% of daily recommended intake
- **Iron**: 6% of daily recommended intake
- **Vitamin A**: 2% of daily recommended intake

Coconut and Matcha Protein Bars are an excellent addition to your healthy snack repertoire. With their combination of wholesome ingredients, these bars offer a great balance of protein, healthy fats, and carbohydrates, making them perfect for post-workout recovery or a mid-afternoon boost. The matcha provides a gentle caffeine lift, while the coconut adds a satisfying texture and flavor. These bars are simple to make and can be customized with your favorite nuts or chocolate chips, allowing you to personalize them to your liking. They are also great for meal prepping, ensuring you always have a nutritious snack on hand. Enjoy the delicious combination of coconut and matcha as you nourish your body and satisfy your taste buds!

Chapter 3

Light & Refreshing Salads

Quinoa and Arugula Salad with Lemon Vinaigrette

Quinoa and Arugula Salad with Lemon Vinaigrette is a refreshing and nutritious dish that perfectly balances the nutty flavor of quinoa with the peppery notes of arugula. This salad is not only vibrant and visually appealing but also packed with essential nutrients, making it an ideal choice for a light lunch or a hearty side dish. Quinoa serves as a complete protein source, providing all nine essential amino acids, while arugula adds a wealth of vitamins A, C, and K, as well as antioxidants. The lemon vinaigrette brings a zesty brightness that enhances the flavors of the salad and adds a touch of acidity to balance the earthiness of the quinoa. Additionally, this salad is versatile; you can easily add seasonal vegetables, nuts, or seeds for extra crunch and nutrition. Whether served on its own or as a side to grilled chicken or fish, this salad is sure to become a staple in your healthy meal rotation. Enjoy it fresh or prepare it in advance for a quick and nutritious meal throughout the week!

Preparation Time

- **Prep Time**: 10 minutes
- **Cook Time**: 15 minutes
- **Total Time**: 25 minutes

Ingredients

- 1 cup quinoa (uncooked)
- 2 cups water or vegetable broth
- 4 cups fresh arugula, washed and dried
- 1 cup cherry tomatoes, halved
- 1/2 cucumber, diced
- 1/4 red onion, thinly sliced
- 1/4 cup feta cheese, crumbled (optional)

- 1/4 cup toasted walnuts or almonds (optional)

Lemon Vinaigrette

- 1/4 cup extra virgin olive oil
- 2 tablespoons fresh lemon juice
- 1 teaspoon Dijon mustard
- 1 teaspoon honey or maple syrup (optional)
- Salt and pepper to taste

Procedure

1. **Cook the Quinoa**: Rinse the quinoa under cold water to remove any bitterness. In a medium saucepan, combine the rinsed quinoa and water or vegetable broth. Bring to a boil, then reduce heat to low, cover, and simmer for about 15 minutes or until the quinoa is fluffy and the liquid is absorbed. Remove from heat and let it sit covered for 5 minutes.

2. **Prepare the Vegetables**: While the quinoa is cooking, wash and prepare the arugula, cherry tomatoes, cucumber, and red onion. Halve the cherry tomatoes, dice the cucumber, and thinly slice the red onion. These colorful vegetables will add freshness and crunch to the salad.

3. **Make the Lemon Vinaigrette**: In a small bowl, whisk together the olive oil, lemon juice, Dijon mustard, and honey (if using). Season with salt and pepper to taste. This vinaigrette will add a bright and zesty flavor to the salad.

4. **Combine Ingredients**: Once the quinoa is cooked and cooled slightly, transfer it to a large mixing bowl. Add the arugula, cherry tomatoes, cucumber, and red onion. If desired, add crumbled feta cheese and toasted nuts for added flavor and texture.

5. **Dress the Salad**: Drizzle the lemon vinaigrette over the salad and toss gently to combine all the ingredients evenly. Ensure the quinoa and vegetables are well coated with the dressing for a balanced flavor.

6. **Taste and Adjust**: Taste the salad and adjust the seasoning if necessary, adding more salt, pepper, or lemon juice to suit your preference. This step allows you to customize the flavors to your liking.

7. **Serve and Enjoy**: Serve the salad immediately or refrigerate it for about 30 minutes to allow the flavors to meld. This salad can be enjoyed fresh or stored in an airtight container in the refrigerator for up to 3 days. It makes for a great make-ahead meal option!

Nutritional Value (per serving, approximately 1 cup)

- **Calories**: ~220
- **Protein**: 7g
- **Carbohydrates**: 27g
- **Fiber**: 4g
- **Fat**: 10g
- **Saturated Fat**: 1.5g
- **Sugar**: 2g
- **Sodium**: 150mg
- **Potassium**: 350mg
- **Vitamin A**: 25% of daily recommended intake
- **Vitamin C**: 15% of daily recommended intake
- **Calcium**: 6% of daily recommended intake
- **Iron**: 10% of daily recommended intake

The *Quinoa and Arugula Salad with Lemon Vinaigrette* is a delightful way to incorporate wholesome ingredients into your diet. Rich in protein and fiber, this salad is both satisfying and nutritious, making it perfect for a light lunch or as a side dish. The combination of quinoa and fresh vegetables offers a variety of textures and flavors, while the lemon vinaigrette brightens the dish and enhances the natural tastes of the ingredients. This recipe is not only easy to prepare but also customizable; feel free to add your favorite vegetables or protein sources to make it your own. With its vibrant colors and delicious taste, this salad is sure to impress at gatherings or become a regular in your meal prep rotation. Enjoy the health benefits and delicious flavors that this salad brings to your table!

Cucumber and Tomato Salad with Avocado & Basil is a refreshing and vibrant dish that celebrates the flavors of fresh summer produce. This salad is light and crisp, making it an ideal choice for a quick lunch or a side dish during barbecues and picnics. The combination of juicy tomatoes, crunchy cucumbers, creamy avocado, and aromatic basil creates a delightful medley of textures and flavors. Avocado adds healthy fats and a smooth richness, while basil brings an herbaceous note that elevates the overall taste of the salad. This recipe is not only simple to prepare but also packed with essential vitamins and antioxidants, making it a nutritious option for any meal. Enjoy this salad chilled for an extra refreshing experience, and feel free to customize it by adding your favorite ingredients, such as feta cheese, olives, or nuts. With its beautiful colors and delicious flavors, this salad is sure to impress both family and guests alike!

Preparation Time

- **Prep Time**: 15 minutes
- **Cook Time**: 0 minutes
- **Total Time**: 15 minutes

Ingredients

- 2 cups cherry tomatoes, halved
- 1 large cucumber, diced
- 1 ripe avocado, diced
- 1/4 cup fresh basil leaves, chopped
- 2 tablespoons extra virgin olive oil
- 1 tablespoon balsamic vinegar (or lemon juice)
- Salt and pepper to taste
- Optional: 1/4 cup red onion, thinly sliced

Procedure

1. **Prepare the Vegetables**: Start by washing the cherry tomatoes and cucumber thoroughly. Halve the cherry tomatoes and dice the cucumber into bite-sized pieces, ensuring they are uniform for even distribution in the salad. If using, thinly slice the red onion for added flavor.

2. **Dice the Avocado**: Cut the avocado in half, remove the pit, and scoop the flesh out with a spoon. Dice the avocado into small cubes and set aside. Be careful not to mash it while handling, as you want to maintain its texture in the salad.

3. **Chop the Basil**: Rinse the fresh basil leaves under cool water and pat them dry with a paper towel. Stack the leaves, roll them up tightly, and slice them into thin ribbons (a technique known as chiffonade). This will release the aromatic oils and enhance the basil's flavor.

4. **Combine the Ingredients**: In a large mixing bowl, combine the halved cherry tomatoes, diced cucumber, diced avocado, and chopped basil. If using, add the sliced red onion for an extra layer of flavor. Gently toss the ingredients together to avoid mashing the avocado.

5. **Make the Dressing**: In a small bowl, whisk together the olive oil, balsamic vinegar (or lemon juice), and a pinch of salt and pepper. This simple dressing will enhance the freshness of the salad without overpowering it.

6. **Dress the Salad**: Drizzle the dressing over the salad and gently toss again to ensure that all ingredients are well coated. Be careful not to stir too vigorously, as you want to keep the avocado intact and avoid mushiness.

7. **Serve Immediately**: Enjoy the salad immediately for the best flavor and texture. If you need to store it, keep it in an airtight container in the refrigerator for up to a day, but note that the avocado may brown slightly. This salad is perfect for summer picnics, barbecues, or as a refreshing side dish!

Nutritional Value (per serving, approximately 1 cup)

- **Calories**: ~180
- **Protein**: 3g
- **Carbohydrates**: 15g
- **Fiber**: 6g

- **Fat**: 12g
- **Saturated Fat**: 1.5g
- **Sugar**: 3g
- **Sodium**: 5mg
- **Potassium**: 350mg
- **Vitamin A**: 15% of daily recommended intake
- **Vitamin C**: 20% of daily recommended intake
- **Calcium**: 2% of daily recommended intake
- **Iron**: 4% of daily recommended intake

Cucumber and Tomato Salad with Avocado & Basil is a delightful way to enjoy fresh ingredients in a nutritious and satisfying manner. This salad is not only visually appealing with its vibrant colors but also offers a burst of flavor in every bite. The combination of creamy avocado, juicy tomatoes, and crunchy cucumbers creates a refreshing texture that is perfect for warm weather. This salad is versatile and can be enjoyed on its own or as a side dish with grilled meats or fish. The use of simple, wholesome ingredients ensures that it is packed with essential nutrients, making it a healthful addition to any meal. Customize the recipe by adding your favorite ingredients or toppings for a personal touch, and enjoy the refreshing flavors of summer all year round!

The *Anti-Inflammatory Power Bowl* is a nutrient-dense dish that brings together a delightful combination of earthy beets, hearty lentils, and nutrient-rich kale. This vibrant bowl is not only visually appealing but also packed with antioxidants, vitamins, and minerals that help combat inflammation and promote overall health. Beets are known for their vibrant color and natural sweetness, while lentils provide a solid source of plant-based protein and fiber. Kale adds a dose of green goodness, being rich in vitamins A, C, and K, and essential minerals like calcium and iron. The bowl can be topped with your choice of nuts, seeds, or a creamy dressing for added texture and flavor. Perfect for lunch or dinner, this power bowl is satisfying and filling while still being light and health-conscious. Enjoy it warm or chilled, making it a versatile option for meal prep or a quick, nourishing meal anytime.

Preparation Time

- **Prep Time**: 15 minutes
- **Cook Time**: 30 minutes
- **Total Time**: 45 minutes

Ingredients

- 1 cup cooked lentils (green or brown)
- 1 medium beet, roasted and diced (or 1 cup canned beets, drained)
- 2 cups fresh kale, stems removed and chopped
- 1/2 cup cherry tomatoes, halved
- 1/4 cup red onion, thinly sliced
- 1 tablespoon olive oil
- 1 tablespoon apple cider vinegar
- Salt and pepper to taste
- Optional toppings: 1/4 cup feta cheese, sliced avocado, or pumpkin seeds

Procedure

1. **Cook the Lentils**: Rinse the lentils under cold water and place them in a saucepan with 2 cups of water. Bring to a boil, then reduce the heat to low, cover, and simmer for about 20-25 minutes, or until the lentils are tender but still hold their shape. Drain any excess water and set aside.

2. **Roast the Beets**: If using fresh beets, preheat your oven to 400°F (200°C). Wrap the beets in aluminum foil and roast for about 30-40 minutes, or until tender. Allow them to cool, peel, and dice them into bite-sized pieces. If using canned beets, simply drain and set them aside.

3. **Prepare the Kale**: In a large mixing bowl, add the chopped kale. Drizzle with olive oil and a pinch of salt, then massage the kale for a minute or two until it begins to soften. This step will enhance the flavor and make the kale easier to digest.

4. **Add Other Ingredients**: To the kale, add the cooked lentils, diced roasted beets, halved cherry tomatoes, and sliced red onion. The combination of these ingredients will create a colorful and nutritious base for the bowl.

5. **Dress the Salad**: In a small bowl, whisk together the apple cider vinegar, salt, and pepper. Pour the dressing over the salad mixture and toss gently to combine, ensuring all ingredients are evenly coated with the dressing.

6. **Taste and Adjust**: Taste the bowl and adjust the seasoning as necessary, adding more salt, pepper, or vinegar to suit your preference. This allows you to customize the flavor to your liking.

7. **Serve and Enjoy**: Serve the Anti-Inflammatory Power Bowl immediately, or refrigerate for about 30 minutes to allow the flavors to meld. Garnish with optional toppings like feta cheese, sliced avocado, or pumpkin seeds for added nutrition and texture. Enjoy this nourishing bowl warm or chilled!

Nutritional Value (per serving, approximately 1 bowl)

- **Calories**: ~350
- **Protein**: 15g
- **Carbohydrates**: 50g

- **Fiber**: 15g
- **Fat**: 10g
- **Saturated Fat**: 2g
- **Sugar**: 5g
- **Sodium**: 150mg
- **Potassium**: 800mg
- **Vitamin A**: 200% of daily recommended intake
- **Vitamin C**: 25% of daily recommended intake
- **Calcium**: 10% of daily recommended intake
- **Iron**: 25% of daily recommended intake

The *Anti-Inflammatory Power Bowl* is a fantastic way to incorporate nutrient-rich ingredients into your diet while enjoying a delicious and satisfying meal. This bowl is not only loaded with flavor but also boasts a wealth of health benefits that help reduce inflammation and support overall wellness. The combination of beets, lentils, and kale provides a variety of textures and tastes that will keep your palate excited. This recipe is highly versatile, allowing you to adapt it with seasonal vegetables or your favorite proteins. Whether you're looking for a quick lunch, a post-workout meal, or a satisfying dinner option, this power bowl delivers on all fronts. Its bright colors and wholesome ingredients will inspire you to prioritize healthy eating without sacrificing flavor. Embrace the nourishing goodness of this Anti-Inflammatory Power Bowl and enjoy the benefits it brings to your health and well-being!

The *Mango and Avocado Salad with Lime Dressing* is a delightful and refreshing dish that combines the tropical sweetness of ripe mangoes with the creamy richness of avocado. This salad is perfect for warm weather, providing a light yet satisfying option that is bursting with flavor and nutrients. Mangoes are rich in vitamins A and C, while avocados contribute healthy fats and fiber, making this salad both nutritious and delicious. The addition of fresh lime dressing brightens the dish and enhances the natural flavors of the ingredients. With vibrant colors and contrasting textures, this salad is not only a feast for the eyes but also a treat for the taste buds. It can be served as a light lunch, a side dish for grilled meats, or a refreshing starter for any meal. Whether enjoyed at a summer barbecue or as a quick snack, this salad is sure to impress with its tropical flair and health benefits.

Preparation Time

- **Prep Time**: 15 minutes
- **Cook Time**: 0 minutes
- **Total Time**: 15 minutes

Ingredients

- 2 ripe mangoes, diced
- 1 ripe avocado, diced
- 1 cup cherry tomatoes, halved
- 1/2 red onion, finely chopped
- 1/4 cup fresh cilantro, chopped
- 1 lime, juiced
- 2 tablespoons extra virgin olive oil
- Salt and pepper to taste
- Optional: 1 jalapeño, finely diced (for heat)

Procedure

1. **Prepare the Ingredients**: Start by washing and preparing all the fresh produce. Dice the mangoes and avocado into bite-sized pieces, halve the cherry tomatoes, and finely chop the red onion and cilantro. If you like a little heat, you can also finely dice the jalapeño.

2. **Mix the Salad**: In a large mixing bowl, combine the diced mangoes, avocado, cherry tomatoes, red onion, and chopped cilantro. Gently toss the ingredients together to ensure they are evenly mixed without mashing the avocado.

3. **Make the Lime Dressing**: In a small bowl, whisk together the lime juice, olive oil, salt, and pepper until well combined. This dressing will add a zesty flavor that complements the sweetness of the mangoes and the creaminess of the avocado.

4. **Dress the Salad**: Drizzle the lime dressing over the salad mixture and toss gently to coat all the ingredients. Be careful not to overmix, as you want to keep the avocado intact and maintain its creamy texture.

5. **Taste and Adjust**: Taste the salad and adjust the seasoning as needed. Add more lime juice, salt, or pepper to suit your preference. This step is crucial for enhancing the flavors of the dish.

6. **Serve Immediately**: Serve the salad immediately to enjoy the freshness of the ingredients. If you need to prepare it ahead of time, consider adding the dressing just before serving to prevent the avocado from browning.

7. **Garnish and Enjoy**: Optionally, garnish the salad with extra cilantro or slices of lime for added presentation. This Mango and Avocado Salad makes a perfect light lunch, a side dish for grilled meats, or a vibrant starter at any gathering!

Nutritional Value (per serving, approximately 1 cup)

- **Calories**: ~220
- **Protein**: 3g
- **Carbohydrates**: 30g
- **Fiber**: 7g

- **Fat**: 10g
- **Saturated Fat**: 1.5g
- **Sugar**: 10g
- **Sodium**: 5mg
- **Potassium**: 500mg
- **Vitamin A**: 20% of daily recommended intake
- **Vitamin C**: 35% of daily recommended intake
- **Calcium**: 2% of daily recommended intake
- **Iron**: 4% of daily recommended intake

The *Mango and Avocado Salad with Lime Dressing* is a celebration of fresh, wholesome ingredients that are both delicious and nutritious. This salad captures the essence of summer with its vibrant colors and tropical flavors, making it a perfect addition to any meal. Rich in essential nutrients, it supports overall health while being easy to prepare and delightful to eat. The balance of sweet, creamy, and zesty elements creates a refreshing dish that appeals to a wide range of palates. Whether enjoyed on its own, served alongside grilled chicken or fish, or as part of a picnic spread, this salad is sure to become a favorite in your repertoire. Embrace the flavors of summer and nourish your body with this delightful Mango and Avocado Salad!

Roasted Sweet Potato & Spinach Salad

The *Roasted Sweet Potato & Spinach Salad* is a wholesome and satisfying dish that combines the earthy sweetness of roasted sweet potatoes with the vibrant freshness of spinach. This salad is perfect for any season, providing a hearty option that is rich in flavor and nutrients. Sweet potatoes are an excellent source of vitamins A and C, fiber, and antioxidants, while spinach is packed with iron, calcium, and vitamins K and E. The addition of crunchy nuts and a zesty dressing elevates the salad, providing a delightful contrast to the tender sweet potatoes. This salad can be enjoyed as a main course or as a side dish, making it a versatile option for lunch or dinner. The combination of warm roasted sweet potatoes and fresh greens creates a comforting yet refreshing meal that is both satisfying and nutritious. Whether you're looking for a nourishing lunch or a colorful side for a dinner party, this salad is sure to impress.

Preparation Time

- **Prep Time**: 15 minutes
- **Cook Time**: 25 minutes
- **Total Time**: 40 minutes

Ingredients

- 2 medium sweet potatoes, peeled and cubed
- 4 cups fresh spinach, washed and dried
- 1/4 cup red onion, thinly sliced
- 1/4 cup walnuts or pecans, roughly chopped
- 2 tablespoons olive oil
- 1 tablespoon maple syrup (optional)
- 1 tablespoon balsamic vinegar
- Salt and pepper to taste
- Optional: 1/4 cup feta cheese, crumbled

Procedure

1. **Preheat the Oven**: Preheat your oven to 400°F (200°C). This ensures that the sweet potatoes roast evenly and develop a delicious caramelized flavor.

2. **Prepare the Sweet Potatoes**: In a large bowl, toss the cubed sweet potatoes with 1 tablespoon of olive oil, salt, and pepper until evenly coated. Spread the sweet potatoes in a single layer on a baking sheet, ensuring they have enough space to roast properly.

3. **Roast the Sweet Potatoes**: Place the baking sheet in the preheated oven and roast the sweet potatoes for 20-25 minutes, or until they are tender and slightly caramelized, flipping them halfway through for even cooking.

4. **Prepare the Dressing**: While the sweet potatoes are roasting, whisk together the remaining 1 tablespoon of olive oil, maple syrup (if using), balsamic vinegar, salt, and pepper in a small bowl. This dressing will add a delightful sweetness and tang to the salad.

5. **Combine the Salad**: In a large mixing bowl, combine the fresh spinach, roasted sweet potatoes, sliced red onion, and chopped nuts. If using feta cheese, add it at this stage for an extra burst of flavor.

6. **Drizzle with Dressing**: Pour the prepared dressing over the salad mixture and gently toss to combine. Be careful not to overmix, as you want to maintain the integrity of the sweet potatoes and spinach.

7. **Serve and Enjoy**: Serve the salad warm or at room temperature. This Roasted Sweet Potato & Spinach Salad makes a perfect main dish or a colorful side for any meal, providing a hearty and nutritious option for any occasion!

Nutritional Value (per serving, approximately 1 cup)

- **Calories**: ~290
- **Protein**: 6g
- **Carbohydrates**: 38g
- **Fiber**: 7g
- **Fat**: 14g
- **Saturated Fat**: 1.5g

- **Sugar**: 6g
- **Sodium**: 150mg
- **Potassium**: 600mg
- **Vitamin A**: 200% of daily recommended intake
- **Vitamin C**: 25% of daily recommended intake
- **Calcium**: 8% of daily recommended intake
- **Iron**: 10% of daily recommended intake

The *Roasted Sweet Potato & Spinach Salad* is a delightful combination of flavors and textures that showcases the natural sweetness of the sweet potatoes and the freshness of the spinach. This salad is not only visually appealing but also offers a wealth of health benefits that support overall well-being. Rich in vitamins and minerals, it makes for a wholesome meal that can be enjoyed at any time of the year. The addition of nuts provides a satisfying crunch, while the dressing ties all the elements together beautifully. This recipe is highly adaptable, allowing you to customize it with seasonal ingredients or your favorite toppings. Whether you're preparing a quick lunch or hosting a gathering, this salad is sure to impress with its vibrant colors and delicious taste. Embrace the nourishing goodness of this Roasted Sweet Potato & Spinach Salad and make it a regular feature in your healthy eating routine!

The *Broccoli & Pomegranate Detox Salad* is a vibrant and nutrient-dense dish that combines the crunchiness of fresh broccoli with the juicy sweetness of pomegranate seeds. This salad is not only refreshing but also packed with detoxifying properties, making it a perfect choice for those looking to boost their health. Broccoli is rich in vitamins C, K, and fiber, while pomegranate seeds provide a wealth of antioxidants and anti-inflammatory benefits. The addition of nuts and a light dressing adds flavor and healthy fats, creating a balanced meal that supports overall well-being. This salad can be enjoyed as a side dish or as a light main course, making it a versatile option for lunch or dinner. With its delightful textures and bright colors, this detox salad is sure to impress anyone who tries it. Perfect for meal prep or a quick weeknight dinner, the *Broccoli & Pomegranate Detox Salad* is a delicious way to nourish your body.

Preparation Time

- **Prep Time**: 15 minutes
- **Cook Time**: 0 minutes
- **Total Time**: 15 minutes

Ingredients

- 2 cups fresh broccoli florets
- 1 cup pomegranate seeds
- 1/4 cup red onion, thinly sliced
- 1/4 cup walnuts or almonds, roughly chopped
- 2 tablespoons extra virgin olive oil
- 1 tablespoon apple cider vinegar
- 1 tablespoon honey or maple syrup (optional)
- Salt and pepper to taste
- Optional: 1/4 cup crumbled feta cheese

Procedure

1. **Prepare the Broccoli**: Start by washing the broccoli florets thoroughly. If desired, you can steam them lightly for 1-2 minutes to enhance their tenderness and bright green color, but this step is optional if you prefer raw broccoli.

2. **Combine the Ingredients**: In a large mixing bowl, combine the fresh broccoli florets, pomegranate seeds, thinly sliced red onion, and chopped nuts. The combination of these ingredients provides a variety of textures and flavors that create an enjoyable eating experience.

3. **Make the Dressing**: In a small bowl, whisk together the olive oil, apple cider vinegar, honey or maple syrup (if using), salt, and pepper. This dressing adds a tangy sweetness that complements the salad beautifully.

4. **Dress the Salad**: Pour the dressing over the salad mixture and gently toss to coat all the ingredients evenly. Be careful not to bruise the pomegranate seeds, as you want them to remain intact and burst with flavor.

5. **Taste and Adjust**: Taste the salad and adjust the seasoning as necessary. Add more salt, pepper, or vinegar according to your preference to enhance the overall flavor of the dish.

6. **Serve Immediately**: Serve the salad immediately to enjoy its freshness and crunch. If preparing ahead of time, consider storing the dressing separately and adding it just before serving to keep the broccoli crisp.

7. **Garnish and Enjoy**: Optionally, garnish the salad with crumbled feta cheese for added creaminess and flavor. This *Broccoli & Pomegranate Detox Salad* makes a nutritious side dish or a light main course, perfect for any occasion!

Nutritional Value (per serving, approximately 1 cup)

- **Calories**: ~180
- **Protein**: 4g
- **Carbohydrates**: 16g
- **Fiber**: 5g
- **Fat**: 12g
- **Saturated Fat**: 1.5g

- **Sugar**: 6g
- **Sodium**: 45mg
- **Potassium**: 450mg
- **Vitamin A**: 20% of daily recommended intake
- **Vitamin C**: 90% of daily recommended intake
- **Calcium**: 6% of daily recommended intake
- **Iron**: 8% of daily recommended intake

The *Broccoli & Pomegranate Detox Salad* is a colorful and nutritious option that supports detoxification while delivering a delicious burst of flavor. This salad showcases the natural sweetness of pomegranates and the crunchiness of fresh broccoli, making it a satisfying dish for any occasion. Rich in antioxidants, vitamins, and minerals, it promotes overall health and well-being. The light dressing enhances the natural flavors of the ingredients without overpowering them, ensuring a delightful eating experience. This recipe is versatile, allowing you to customize it with additional ingredients like grilled chicken, quinoa, or other seasonal vegetables. Whether enjoyed as a refreshing lunch or served alongside a main course, this detox salad is sure to become a staple in your healthy eating routine. Enjoy the vibrant flavors and health benefits of this *Broccoli & Pomegranate Detox Salad* as a nourishing addition to your meals!

The *Chickpea and Turmeric Couscous Salad* is a vibrant, protein-packed dish that combines the nutty flavors of couscous with the earthy richness of turmeric and the hearty texture of chickpeas. This salad is not only quick and easy to prepare, but it is also loaded with nutrients, making it a perfect option for a satisfying lunch or a light dinner. Chickpeas are a fantastic source of plant-based protein and fiber, while turmeric is celebrated for its anti-inflammatory properties and bright yellow hue. The addition of fresh vegetables and a zesty dressing elevates the salad, bringing a delightful contrast of flavors and textures. This dish can be served warm or cold, making it versatile for any occasion. The *Chickpea and Turmeric Couscous Salad* is also ideal for meal prep, as it holds well in the refrigerator, allowing the flavors to meld together over time. Whether enjoyed as a main course or a side dish, this salad is a delicious way to incorporate healthy ingredients into your diet.

Preparation Time

- **Prep Time**: 15 minutes
- **Cook Time**: 10 minutes
- **Total Time**: 25 minutes

Ingredients

- 1 cup couscous
- 1 1/2 cups vegetable broth (or water)
- 1 can (15 oz) chickpeas, drained and rinsed
- 1 teaspoon turmeric powder
- 1/2 cup cucumber, diced
- 1/2 cup cherry tomatoes, halved
- 1/4 cup red onion, finely chopped
- 1/4 cup fresh parsley or cilantro, chopped
- 2 tablespoons olive oil
- 1 tablespoon lemon juice
- Salt and pepper to taste
- Optional: 1/4 cup feta cheese, crumbled

Procedure

1. **Prepare the Couscous**: In a medium saucepan, bring the vegetable broth (or water) to a boil. Once boiling, stir in the couscous and turmeric powder. Remove from heat, cover, and let it sit for about 5 minutes until the couscous absorbs the liquid.
2. **Fluff the Couscous**: After the couscous has absorbed the liquid, fluff it with a fork to separate the grains. Set aside to cool slightly while you prepare the other ingredients.
3. **Combine the Ingredients**: In a large mixing bowl, combine the cooked couscous, chickpeas, diced cucumber, cherry tomatoes, red onion, and chopped parsley or cilantro. This mixture of ingredients creates a colorful and nutritious salad that is both satisfying and refreshing.
4. **Make the Dressing**: In a small bowl, whisk together the olive oil, lemon juice, salt, and pepper until well combined. This dressing will add a bright and zesty flavor to the salad, complementing the earthiness of the turmeric and chickpeas.
5. **Dress the Salad**: Pour the dressing over the couscous mixture and toss gently to combine, ensuring all ingredients are evenly coated. Be careful not to mash the chickpeas; you want to maintain their texture in the salad.
6. **Taste and Adjust**: Taste the salad and adjust the seasoning if needed. Add more salt, pepper, or lemon juice to enhance the flavors to your liking.
7. **Serve and Enjoy**: Serve the salad warm or cold, and if desired, sprinkle with crumbled feta cheese for an extra layer of flavor. This *Chickpea and Turmeric Couscous Salad* makes a delightful main dish or side dish, perfect for any occasion!

Nutritional Value (per serving, approximately 1 cup)

- **Calories**: ~250
- **Protein**: 9g
- **Carbohydrates**: 38g
- **Fiber**: 6g

- **Fat**: 7g
- **Saturated Fat**: 1g
- **Sugar**: 3g
- **Sodium**: 250mg
- **Potassium**: 500mg
- **Vitamin A**: 10% of daily recommended intake
- **Vitamin C**: 15% of daily recommended intake
- **Calcium**: 4% of daily recommended intake
- **Iron**: 15% of daily recommended intake

The *Chickpea and Turmeric Couscous Salad* is a delightful blend of flavors and textures, offering a healthy and filling meal option. Rich in nutrients and easy to prepare, this salad is perfect for busy weeknights or meal prep, allowing you to enjoy nutritious food without spending hours in the kitchen. The vibrant colors of the ingredients make it visually appealing, while the combination of chickpeas, turmeric, and fresh vegetables provides an abundance of health benefits. With its versatility, you can easily customize this salad by adding your favorite ingredients, such as bell peppers, avocado, or other seasonal vegetables. Whether served as a hearty lunch or a side dish at a gathering, this salad is sure to please both the palate and the body. Enjoy the deliciousness and nourishment of the *Chickpea and Turmeric Couscous Salad* as a staple in your healthy eating repertoire!

Watermelon and Feta Anti-Inflammatory Salad

The *Watermelon and Feta Anti-Inflammatory Salad* is a refreshing and vibrant dish that beautifully balances sweet and savory flavors while providing a wealth of health benefits. This salad is perfect for hot summer days or as a light appetizer at any gathering. Watermelon is not only hydrating but also rich in antioxidants like lycopene, which has been shown to have anti-inflammatory properties. The creamy feta cheese adds a delightful contrast to the sweetness of the watermelon, while fresh mint and a splash of lime juice elevate the overall flavor profile. This dish is not only visually appealing, with its striking colors, but it is also incredibly easy to prepare. The *Watermelon and Feta Anti-Inflammatory Salad* can be made in just a few minutes, making it an excellent option for quick meals or potlucks. With its refreshing taste and nutritious ingredients, this salad is a delicious way to support a healthy diet.

Preparation Time

- **Prep Time**: 10 minutes
- **Cook Time**: 0 minutes
- **Total Time**: 10 minutes

Ingredients

- 4 cups watermelon, cubed (seedless)
- 1 cup feta cheese, crumbled
- 1/4 cup fresh mint leaves, chopped
- 2 tablespoons extra virgin olive oil
- 1 tablespoon lime juice
- Salt and pepper to taste
- Optional: 1/4 cup red onion, thinly sliced

Procedure

1. **Prepare the Watermelon**: Start by cutting the seedless watermelon into bite-sized cubes. If you're using a whole watermelon, slice it in half and scoop out the flesh with a melon baller or a spoon for a fun presentation.

2. **Combine the Ingredients**: In a large mixing bowl, combine the cubed watermelon, crumbled feta cheese, and chopped fresh mint leaves. If you enjoy a bit of onion flavor, you can add the thinly sliced red onion at this stage for an extra layer of taste.

3. **Make the Dressing**: In a small bowl, whisk together the extra virgin olive oil, lime juice, salt, and pepper until well combined. This dressing adds a light and zesty touch to the salad, enhancing the natural flavors of the ingredients.

4. **Dress the Salad**: Drizzle the dressing over the watermelon mixture and gently toss everything together to combine, ensuring that the feta cheese remains intact while the watermelon is coated with the dressing.

5. **Taste and Adjust**: Taste the salad and adjust the seasoning if necessary. You may want to add a pinch more salt, pepper, or lime juice to enhance the flavors according to your preference.

6. **Chill and Serve**: For an extra refreshing experience, you can chill the salad in the refrigerator for about 15 minutes before serving. This allows the flavors to meld together beautifully.

7. **Garnish and Enjoy**: Serve the *Watermelon and Feta Anti-Inflammatory Salad* immediately, garnished with additional mint leaves if desired. This salad is perfect as a light lunch, a side dish at a barbecue, or a refreshing appetizer at any gathering!

Nutritional Value (per serving, approximately 1 cup)

- **Calories**: ~150
- **Protein**: 5g
- **Carbohydrates**: 14g
- **Fiber**: 1g
- **Fat**: 9g

- **Saturated Fat**: 4g
- **Sugar**: 6g
- **Sodium**: 300mg
- **Potassium**: 250mg
- **Vitamin A**: 10% of daily recommended intake
- **Vitamin C**: 20% of daily recommended intake
- **Calcium**: 10% of daily recommended intake
- **Iron**: 4% of daily recommended intake

The *Watermelon and Feta Anti-Inflammatory Salad* is a delightful mix of flavors that not only satisfies your taste buds but also nourishes your body. The refreshing watermelon provides hydration and essential nutrients, while the feta cheese contributes protein and a creamy texture. This salad is versatile enough to be enjoyed at picnics, barbecues, or as a light lunch during hot days. Its bright colors and appealing presentation make it an eye-catching dish that's sure to impress guests. Whether you're seeking a healthy side dish or a satisfying main course, this salad is an excellent choice that embodies the spirit of summertime eating. Enjoy the delicious and nourishing benefits of this *Watermelon and Feta Anti-Inflammatory Salad* as a staple in your healthy meal rotation!

Chapter 4

Satisfying Soups & Stews

Ginger and Carrot Soup

The *Ginger and Carrot Soup* is a comforting and aromatic dish that combines the natural sweetness of carrots with the zesty kick of fresh ginger. This soup is not only delicious but also offers numerous health benefits, thanks to the anti-inflammatory properties of ginger and the rich vitamin A content in carrots. Perfect for chilly evenings or as a light lunch, this soup is creamy, velvety, and satisfying without being heavy. The vibrant orange color of the soup is visually appealing, and it can be served warm or chilled, making it a versatile option for any season. This recipe is simple to prepare and can be made in under an hour, making it an ideal choice for busy weeknights. Additionally, the soup can easily be made in larger batches and stored for meal prep, allowing the flavors to deepen over time. Enjoy this *Ginger and Carrot Soup* as a nourishing dish that warms the soul and delights the palate.

Preparation Time

- **Prep Time**: 10 minutes
- **Cook Time**: 30 minutes
- **Total Time**: 40 minutes

Ingredients

- 1 tablespoon olive oil
- 1 medium onion, chopped
- 2 cloves garlic, minced
- 1 tablespoon fresh ginger, grated
- 4 cups carrots, peeled and sliced
- 4 cups vegetable broth
- 1 teaspoon ground cumin
- Salt and pepper to taste

- Optional: 1 cup coconut milk for creaminess
- Garnish: Fresh cilantro or parsley, for serving

Procedure

1. **Sauté the Aromatics**: In a large pot, heat the olive oil over medium heat. Add the chopped onion and sauté until translucent, about 5 minutes. Then, stir in the minced garlic and grated ginger, cooking for another 2 minutes until fragrant.
2. **Add Carrots**: Add the sliced carrots to the pot and stir to combine with the aromatics. Cook for about 5 minutes, allowing the carrots to soften slightly.
3. **Pour in the Broth**: Add the vegetable broth and ground cumin to the pot, bringing the mixture to a boil. Once boiling, reduce the heat to a simmer, cover, and let it cook for about 20 minutes or until the carrots are tender.
4. **Blend the Soup**: Remove the pot from heat and let it cool slightly. Using an immersion blender, blend the soup until smooth and creamy. Alternatively, you can transfer the soup to a countertop blender in batches, ensuring to let the steam escape.
5. **Add Coconut Milk (Optional)**: If using, stir in the coconut milk to the blended soup for added creaminess. Mix well to combine and adjust the consistency with additional broth or water if needed.
6. **Season to Taste**: Taste the soup and season with salt and pepper as desired. You can also add more ground cumin for additional flavor if you prefer.
7. **Serve and Garnish**: Ladle the *Ginger and Carrot Soup* into bowls and garnish with fresh cilantro or parsley before serving. This soup is delicious served warm, and you can enjoy it with crusty bread or as a standalone dish.

Nutritional Value (per serving, approximately 1 cup)

- **Calories**: ~150
- **Protein**: 3g
- **Carbohydrates**: 25g
- **Fiber**: 4g

- **Fat**: 5g
- **Saturated Fat**: 1g
- **Sugar**: 6g
- **Sodium**: 350mg
- **Potassium**: 450mg
- **Vitamin A**: 180% of daily recommended intake
- **Vitamin C**: 10% of daily recommended intake
- **Calcium**: 4% of daily recommended intake
- **Iron**: 6% of daily recommended intake

The *Ginger and Carrot Soup* is a wholesome and flavorful dish that nourishes both body and soul. With its vibrant color and comforting flavors, this soup is perfect for cozy evenings and can be easily adapted to suit your taste preferences. The combination of ginger and carrots not only adds depth to the flavor but also provides numerous health benefits, making it an excellent addition to any diet. The soup's creamy texture, enhanced by the optional coconut milk, makes it satisfying without being heavy. Whether you're looking for a light lunch, a starter for dinner, or a quick meal prep option, this soup fits the bill. Enjoy the warmth and nourishment of this *Ginger and Carrot Soup* as a delightful part of your culinary repertoire!

Hearty Lentil and Vegetable Stew

The *Hearty Lentil and Vegetable Stew* is a nourishing and satisfying dish that packs a punch of flavors while providing a wealth of nutrients. This stew is perfect for cold weather, offering warmth and comfort in every bowl. Lentils are a fantastic source of plant-based protein, fiber, and essential vitamins and minerals, making them a staple in many healthy diets. Coupled with a medley of colorful vegetables like carrots, potatoes, and spinach, this stew not only delights the taste buds but also supports overall health. The rich broth, infused with aromatic herbs and spices, enhances the depth of flavor, making this stew a favorite among both vegetarians and meat-lovers alike. This recipe is incredibly versatile, allowing you to use whatever vegetables you have on hand or prefer. With minimal prep and cook time, the *Hearty Lentil and Vegetable Stew* is an ideal choice for busy weeknights or meal prep, providing hearty servings that can be enjoyed throughout the week.

Preparation Time

- **Prep Time**: 15 minutes
- **Cook Time**: 30 minutes
- **Total Time**: 45 minutes

Ingredients

- 1 tablespoon olive oil
- 1 medium onion, chopped
- 2 cloves garlic, minced
- 2 medium carrots, diced
- 1 medium potato, diced
- 1 cup celery, diced
- 1 cup spinach, chopped (or any leafy greens)
- 1 cup dried green or brown lentils, rinsed
- 6 cups vegetable broth
- 1 teaspoon ground cumin
- 1 teaspoon dried thyme
- 1 bay leaf

- Salt and pepper to taste
- Optional: 1 can (14.5 oz) diced tomatoes (with juices)
- Garnish: Fresh parsley, chopped

Procedure

1. **Sauté the Aromatics**: In a large pot, heat the olive oil over medium heat. Add the chopped onion and sauté until translucent, about 5 minutes. Stir in the minced garlic and cook for another minute until fragrant, which will form a flavorful base for the stew.
2. **Add the Vegetables**: Incorporate the diced carrots, potato, and celery into the pot. Cook for 5–7 minutes, stirring occasionally, until the vegetables begin to soften and the aromas blend together beautifully.
3. **Add the Lentils and Broth**: Stir in the rinsed lentils, vegetable broth, ground cumin, dried thyme, and bay leaf. If using, add the diced tomatoes along with their juices for added richness and flavor. Bring the mixture to a boil.
4. **Simmer the Stew**: Once boiling, reduce the heat to low and cover the pot. Let the stew simmer for about 25–30 minutes or until the lentils are tender. Stir occasionally to prevent sticking and ensure even cooking.
5. **Add the Greens**: When the lentils are tender, stir in the chopped spinach or any leafy greens of your choice. Allow the stew to cook for an additional 5 minutes until the greens are wilted and vibrant.
6. **Season to Taste**: Taste the stew and adjust the seasoning with salt and pepper as desired. This is also a great time to remove the bay leaf, as it's no longer needed.
7. **Serve and Garnish**: Ladle the *Hearty Lentil and Vegetable Stew* into bowls and garnish with fresh chopped parsley before serving. This stew is perfect on its own or served with crusty bread for a complete meal!

Nutritional Value (per serving, approximately 1 cup)

- **Calories**: ~220
- **Protein**: 12g
- **Carbohydrates**: 35g

- **Fiber**: 9g
- **Fat**: 5g
- **Saturated Fat**: 1g
- **Sugar**: 3g
- **Sodium**: 400mg
- **Potassium**: 600mg
- **Vitamin A**: 80% of daily recommended intake
- **Vitamin C**: 15% of daily recommended intake
- **Calcium**: 6% of daily recommended intake
- **Iron**: 15% of daily recommended intake

The *Hearty Lentil and Vegetable Stew* is a wholesome and satisfying meal that nourishes both body and spirit. Packed with protein, fiber, and a range of vitamins and minerals, this stew is a perfect choice for those looking to eat healthily without sacrificing flavor. The combination of lentils and assorted vegetables creates a rich and hearty texture that is truly comforting, making it an ideal option for meal prep. Whether enjoyed on a chilly evening or as a hearty lunch, this stew offers versatility in flavor and ingredients, allowing for personal customization. With its delightful balance of nutrients and flavors, the *Hearty Lentil and Vegetable Stew* is sure to become a staple in your healthy cooking repertoire. Enjoy the warmth and comfort of this nourishing dish that is as delightful as it is nutritious!

The *Turmeric Butternut Squash Soup* is a vibrant and flavorful dish that beautifully combines the natural sweetness of butternut squash with the warm, earthy notes of turmeric. This soup is not only comforting but also brimming with health benefits, thanks to the anti-inflammatory properties of turmeric and the rich vitamins and minerals found in squash. Ideal for a cozy dinner or a nutritious lunch, this creamy soup can be enjoyed warm or chilled, making it versatile for any season. The addition of coconut milk adds a delightful creaminess, while the spices elevate the flavor profile, making it a favorite among both plant-based eaters and soup lovers alike. Easy to prepare, this recipe requires minimal ingredients and can be made in under an hour, perfect for busy weeknights or meal prep. Garnished with fresh herbs or a drizzle of coconut cream, the *Turmeric Butternut Squash Soup* is not only delicious but also visually appealing. This soup is a wonderful way to nourish your body while indulging in comforting flavors.

Preparation Time

- **Prep Time**: 10 minutes
- **Cook Time**: 30 minutes
- **Total Time**: 40 minutes

Ingredients

- 1 tablespoon olive oil
- 1 medium onion, chopped
- 2 cloves garlic, minced
- 1 tablespoon fresh ginger, grated
- 1 medium butternut squash, peeled and diced (about 4 cups)
- 4 cups vegetable broth
- 1 teaspoon ground turmeric
- 1 teaspoon ground cumin
- 1 can (14 oz) coconut milk
- Salt and pepper to taste
- Optional: Fresh cilantro or parsley for garnish

Procedure

1. **Sauté the Aromatics**: In a large pot, heat the olive oil over medium heat. Add the chopped onion and sauté for about 5 minutes until translucent. Stir in the minced garlic and grated ginger, cooking for an additional minute until fragrant, which forms a flavorful base for the soup.

2. **Add Butternut Squash**: Incorporate the diced butternut squash into the pot and stir to combine with the aromatics. Cook for about 5 minutes, allowing the squash to soften slightly and absorb the flavors.

3. **Add Broth and Spices**: Pour in the vegetable broth and add the ground turmeric and cumin. Bring the mixture to a boil, then reduce the heat to a simmer, covering the pot. Let it simmer for about 20–25 minutes or until the squash is tender.

4. **Blend the Soup**: Once the squash is tender, remove the pot from heat and let it cool slightly. Using an immersion blender, blend the soup until smooth and creamy. Alternatively, you can transfer the soup in batches to a countertop blender, ensuring steam can escape.

5. **Stir in Coconut Milk**: After blending, return the pot to low heat and stir in the coconut milk. This adds creaminess and a hint of sweetness to the soup, enhancing the overall flavor.

6. **Season to Taste**: Taste the soup and adjust the seasoning with salt and pepper as needed. This is also the time to add any additional turmeric or spices to suit your preference.

7. **Serve and Garnish**: Ladle the *Turmeric Butternut Squash Soup* into bowls and garnish with fresh cilantro or parsley if desired. This soup is delicious served warm, and you can accompany it with crusty bread or a light salad for a complete meal.

Nutritional Value (per serving, approximately 1 cup)

- **Calories**: ~180
- **Protein**: 3g
- **Carbohydrates**: 22g
- **Fiber**: 4g
- **Fat**: 9g
- **Saturated Fat**: 6g
- **Sugar**: 2g

- **Sodium**: 300mg
- **Potassium**: 450mg
- **Vitamin A**: 150% of daily recommended intake
- **Vitamin C**: 15% of daily recommended intake
- **Calcium**: 6% of daily recommended intake
- **Iron**: 8% of daily recommended intake

The *Turmeric Butternut Squash Soup* is a delightful blend of flavors that not only satisfies your palate but also nourishes your body. Packed with nutrients and antioxidants, this soup is a great addition to your healthy meal rotation. The vibrant color and creamy texture make it a visually appealing dish, perfect for impressing guests or enjoying as a cozy dinner. With its comforting warmth and rich flavors, this soup is a wonderful way to savor the benefits of seasonal produce while embracing the healthful qualities of turmeric. Whether you're seeking a light lunch, a warm appetizer, or a simple dinner, the *Turmeric Butternut Squash Soup* is a fantastic choice that delivers both taste and nutrition. Enjoy this heartwarming soup as a nourishing way to brighten up your day!

The *Mushroom and Barley Soup* is a hearty, flavorful dish that combines the earthiness of mushrooms with the nutty taste of barley, creating a comforting meal perfect for any time of year. This soup is packed with nutrition, offering a rich source of fiber, protein, and various vitamins and minerals, making it an excellent choice for a wholesome, plant-based meal. The mushrooms add umami depth to the broth, while the barley provides a satisfying chewiness, making each spoonful a delight. Infused with aromatic herbs and spices, this soup fills the kitchen with warmth and inviting aromas, perfect for chilly evenings or casual family dinners. The simplicity of this recipe makes it easy to prepare, and it can be made in under an hour, allowing you to enjoy a nutritious meal without spending all day in the kitchen. Additionally, this soup can be made in large batches and freezes well, making it an ideal option for meal prepping. Enjoy the *Mushroom and Barley Soup* as a standalone dish or pair it with a fresh salad or crusty bread for a complete and nourishing meal.

Preparation Time

- **Prep Time**: 10 minutes
- **Cook Time**: 30 minutes
- **Total Time**: 40 minutes

Ingredients

- 1 tablespoon olive oil
- 1 medium onion, chopped
- 2 cloves garlic, minced
- 2 cups mushrooms, sliced (such as cremini or button mushrooms)
- 1 cup carrots, diced
- 1 cup celery, diced
- 1 cup barley, rinsed
- 6 cups vegetable broth
- 1 teaspoon dried thyme
- 1 teaspoon dried rosemary
- Salt and pepper to taste

- Optional: Fresh parsley for garnish

Procedure

1. **Sauté the Aromatics**: In a large pot, heat the olive oil over medium heat. Add the chopped onion and sauté for about 5 minutes until softened and translucent. Stir in the minced garlic and cook for an additional minute until fragrant, forming a flavorful base for the soup.
2. **Add the Vegetables**: Incorporate the sliced mushrooms, diced carrots, and diced celery into the pot. Cook for about 5–7 minutes, stirring occasionally, until the mushrooms are tender and have released their moisture.
3. **Add Barley and Broth**: Stir in the rinsed barley, then pour in the vegetable broth. Add the dried thyme and rosemary for aromatic flavor. Bring the mixture to a boil.
4. **Simmer the Soup**: Once boiling, reduce the heat to low and cover the pot. Let the soup simmer for about 25 minutes or until the barley is tender and the flavors have melded beautifully. Stir occasionally to prevent sticking.
5. **Season to Taste**: After the barley has cooked, taste the soup and adjust the seasoning with salt and pepper as needed. This is a great time to add additional herbs if you desire a more intense flavor.
6. **Garnish and Serve**: Remove the pot from heat and let the soup cool slightly before serving. Ladle the *Mushroom and Barley Soup* into bowls and garnish with fresh parsley if desired for a touch of color and freshness.
7. **Enjoy**: Serve the soup warm, either on its own or with a side of crusty bread or a fresh salad for a complete meal.

Nutritional Value (per serving, approximately 1 cup)

- **Calories**: ~190
- **Protein**: 6g
- **Carbohydrates**: 36g
- **Fiber**: 8g
- **Fat**: 4g
- **Saturated Fat**: 0.5g

- **Sugar**: 3g
- **Sodium**: 300mg
- **Potassium**: 500mg
- **Vitamin A**: 70% of daily recommended intake
- **Vitamin C**: 5% of daily recommended intake
- **Calcium**: 2% of daily recommended intake
- **Iron**: 10% of daily recommended intake

The *Mushroom and Barley Soup* is a comforting dish that satisfies both hunger and taste. Loaded with nutritious ingredients, this soup not only provides health benefits but also warms the soul. The combination of mushrooms and barley creates a rich and hearty texture, while the herbs enhance the overall flavor profile. Perfect for meal prep, this soup can be made in large batches and stored in the refrigerator or freezer for later enjoyment. Whether served as a starter, main course, or a light meal, the *Mushroom and Barley Soup* is a delicious way to embrace wholesome eating. With its hearty ingredients and warm flavors, this soup is sure to become a staple in your kitchen, bringing comfort and nourishment to every bowl!

The *Spicy Black Bean Soup* is a vibrant and hearty dish that combines the richness of black beans with a kick of spice, making it an ideal choice for those who love bold flavors. This soup is not only satisfying but also packed with protein and fiber, providing a nutritious and filling meal. Black beans are known for their numerous health benefits, including being an excellent source of antioxidants, vitamins, and minerals. This recipe is simple to prepare and can be made in under an hour, perfect for busy weeknights or meal prep. The combination of spices, including cumin and chili powder, infuses the soup with warmth and depth, while the addition of fresh lime juice adds a refreshing brightness. Whether enjoyed on its own or topped with your favorite garnishes, such as avocado, cilantro, or tortilla chips, the *Spicy Black Bean Soup* is sure to please. This soup also freezes well, making it a convenient option for quick meals in the future.

Preparation Time

- **Prep Time**: 10 minutes
- **Cook Time**: 30 minutes
- **Total Time**: 40 minutes

Ingredients

- 1 tablespoon olive oil
- 1 medium onion, chopped
- 2 cloves garlic, minced
- 1 bell pepper, chopped (any color)
- 1 teaspoon ground cumin
- 1 teaspoon chili powder
- 1/2 teaspoon smoked paprika
- 2 cans (15 oz each) black beans, rinsed and drained
- 4 cups vegetable broth
- 1 can (14.5 oz) diced tomatoes (with juices)
- Salt and pepper to taste
- Optional toppings: Fresh cilantro, avocado, lime wedges, or tortilla chips

Procedure

1. **Sauté the Aromatics**: In a large pot, heat the olive oil over medium heat. Add the chopped onion and sauté for about 5 minutes until it becomes translucent and fragrant. Stir in the minced garlic and chopped bell pepper, cooking for an additional 3–4 minutes until the vegetables soften.

2. **Add the Spices**: Sprinkle in the ground cumin, chili powder, and smoked paprika. Stir the mixture for about a minute, allowing the spices to toast and release their aromatic flavors, which will enhance the overall taste of the soup.

3. **Incorporate the Beans and Broth**: Add the rinsed and drained black beans, diced tomatoes (with their juices), and vegetable broth to the pot. Stir to combine all the ingredients, bringing the mixture to a gentle boil.

4. **Simmer the Soup**: Once boiling, reduce the heat to low and let the soup simmer for about 20 minutes. This allows the flavors to meld together beautifully and the soup to thicken slightly. Stir occasionally to prevent sticking and ensure even cooking.

5. **Blend for Creaminess**: After simmering, you can choose to blend the soup for a creamier texture. Using an immersion blender, blend about half of the soup, or transfer half to a countertop blender and blend until smooth. Alternatively, you can leave it chunky for more texture.

6. **Season to Taste**: Return the blended soup to the pot (if blended separately) and adjust the seasoning with salt and pepper to taste. For an extra kick, you can also add a few dashes of hot sauce if desired.

7. **Serve and Garnish**: Ladle the *Spicy Black Bean Soup* into bowls and top with fresh cilantro, diced avocado, and lime wedges for added flavor and brightness. Serve with tortilla chips for a crunchy side, if desired.

Nutritional Value (per serving, approximately 1 cup)

- **Calories**: ~210
- **Protein**: 10g
- **Carbohydrates**: 35g
- **Fiber**: 10g

- **Fat**: 4g

- **Saturated Fat**: 0.5g

- **Sugar**: 2g

- **Sodium**: 350mg

- **Potassium**: 500mg

- **Vitamin A**: 15% of daily recommended intake

- **Vitamin C**: 25% of daily recommended intake

- **Calcium**: 6% of daily recommended intake

- **Iron**: 15% of daily recommended intake

The *Spicy Black Bean Soup* is a delightful fusion of flavor and nutrition, making it a wonderful addition to your meal repertoire. Rich in plant-based protein and fiber, this soup is both filling and healthy, perfect for a quick lunch or a hearty dinner. The depth of flavor achieved through simple spices elevates this soup, transforming basic ingredients into a satisfying dish. It's versatile, allowing you to customize toppings and add-ins to suit your personal preferences. Whether enjoyed on a chilly day or as a light meal any time of year, the *Spicy Black Bean Soup* is sure to warm your soul. Enjoy this nourishing soup as a go-to recipe for comfort, flavor, and wellness!

The *Coconut Milk and Lemongrass Soup* is a fragrant and flavorful dish that showcases the aromatic essence of lemongrass and the creamy richness of coconut milk. This soup is inspired by Southeast Asian cuisine, offering a delightful balance of sweet, savory, and tangy flavors. Lemongrass adds a unique citrusy note that elevates the dish, while coconut milk contributes a smooth, velvety texture, making each spoonful a comforting experience. Packed with fresh vegetables and herbs, this soup is not only delicious but also loaded with nutrients, making it a perfect choice for a light yet satisfying meal. The simplicity of this recipe allows for quick preparation, making it an ideal option for busy weeknights or when you're craving something exotic. This soup can easily be customized by adding proteins like tofu, chicken, or shrimp, depending on your dietary preferences. Enjoy the *Coconut Milk and Lemongrass Soup* as a standalone dish or paired with rice or noodles for a complete meal.

Preparation Time

- **Prep Time**: 10 minutes
- **Cook Time**: 20 minutes
- **Total Time**: 30 minutes

Ingredients

- 1 tablespoon coconut oil
- 1 medium onion, thinly sliced
- 2 cloves garlic, minced
- 1 stalk lemongrass, trimmed and smashed
- 1 tablespoon fresh ginger, grated
- 2 cups vegetable broth
- 1 can (14 oz) coconut milk
- 1 cup mushrooms, sliced (such as shiitake or button)
- 1 cup bell pepper, thinly sliced
- 1 cup baby spinach or kale
- 2 tablespoons soy sauce or tamari
- Juice of 1 lime

- Salt and pepper to taste
- Optional garnish: Fresh cilantro, lime wedges, and sliced chili peppers

Procedure

1. **Sauté the Aromatics**: In a large pot, heat the coconut oil over medium heat. Add the sliced onion and sauté for about 5 minutes until softened and translucent. Stir in the minced garlic, grated ginger, and smashed lemongrass, cooking for an additional minute until fragrant.
2. **Add the Broth**: Pour in the vegetable broth, scraping up any bits stuck to the bottom of the pot. Bring the mixture to a gentle boil, allowing the flavors from the lemongrass and spices to infuse the broth.
3. **Incorporate the Coconut Milk**: Reduce the heat and stir in the coconut milk, mixing well to combine with the broth. Allow the mixture to simmer for a few minutes to thicken slightly and meld the flavors.
4. **Add Vegetables**: Stir in the sliced mushrooms and bell pepper, cooking for another 5 minutes until the vegetables are tender but still crisp.
5. **Finish with Greens**: Add the baby spinach or kale and cook for an additional 2 minutes until wilted. This adds a pop of color and additional nutrients to the soup.
6. **Season and Serve**: Remove the pot from heat and discard the lemongrass stalk. Stir in the soy sauce and lime juice, adjusting the seasoning with salt and pepper to taste.
7. **Garnish and Enjoy**: Ladle the *Coconut Milk and Lemongrass Soup* into bowls and garnish with fresh cilantro, lime wedges, and sliced chili peppers if desired. Serve warm and enjoy the vibrant flavors!

Nutritional Value (per serving, approximately 1 cup)

- **Calories**: ~180
- **Protein**: 3g
- **Carbohydrates**: 14g
- **Fiber**: 2g
- **Fat**: 13g
- **Saturated Fat**: 11g

- **Sugar**: 2g
- **Sodium**: 400mg
- **Potassium**: 350mg
- **Vitamin A**: 15% of daily recommended intake
- **Vitamin C**: 20% of daily recommended intake
- **Calcium**: 4% of daily recommended intake
- **Iron**: 6% of daily recommended intake

The *Coconut Milk and Lemongrass Soup* is a delightful dish that transports you to the tropical flavors of Southeast Asia with every bite. The aromatic notes of lemongrass combined with the creaminess of coconut milk create a soothing and flavorful experience that warms the heart and nourishes the body. This versatile soup is easy to prepare and can be customized with your choice of vegetables or proteins, making it suitable for various dietary needs. The balance of spices and the freshness of herbs make it a vibrant and appealing addition to your meal repertoire. Perfect for a light lunch or as a starter for dinner, this soup is sure to impress your family and friends. Enjoy the refreshing flavors of the *Coconut Milk and Lemongrass Soup* as a quick and nourishing meal that brings comfort and joy to your table!

Red Lentil Dhal with Turmeric and Ginger is a comforting, nutritious dish rooted in Indian cuisine, known for its rich flavors and vibrant colors. This wholesome meal features red lentils, which cook quickly and become wonderfully creamy when simmered, creating a satisfying base that is both hearty and nourishing. The addition of turmeric and ginger not only enhances the flavor profile but also infuses the dish with anti-inflammatory properties, making it a healthful choice. This dhal is typically served with rice or flatbreads, but it can also be enjoyed on its own as a warming soup. Quick to prepare, it is an excellent option for busy weeknights or when you want a simple yet fulfilling meal. This recipe is also incredibly versatile, allowing for easy adaptations based on available ingredients or personal preferences. Topped with fresh cilantro or a squeeze of lime, *Red Lentil Dhal* becomes a delightful dish that is sure to satisfy your taste buds while nourishing your body.

Preparation Time

- **Prep Time**: 10 minutes
- **Cook Time**: 30 minutes
- **Total Time**: 40 minutes

Ingredients

- 1 tablespoon coconut oil or olive oil
- 1 medium onion, finely chopped
- 2 cloves garlic, minced
- 1-inch piece of fresh ginger, grated
- 1 teaspoon ground turmeric
- 1 teaspoon ground cumin
- 1 teaspoon ground coriander
- 1 cup red lentils, rinsed and drained
- 4 cups vegetable broth or water
- 1 can (14 oz) coconut milk (optional for creaminess)
- Salt and pepper to taste

- Fresh cilantro for garnish
- Optional: Lime wedges for serving

Procedure

1. **Sauté the Aromatics**: In a large pot, heat the coconut oil or olive oil over medium heat. Add the chopped onion and sauté for about 5 minutes until it becomes translucent and soft. Stir in the minced garlic and grated ginger, cooking for an additional 1-2 minutes until fragrant.
2. **Add the Spices**: Sprinkle in the ground turmeric, cumin, and coriander, stirring to combine. Allow the spices to toast for about a minute, releasing their flavors and aromas into the pot.
3. **Incorporate the Lentils**: Add the rinsed red lentils to the pot, stirring to coat them with the spice mixture. This helps to enhance their flavor as they cook.
4. **Pour in the Liquid**: Pour in the vegetable broth or water, bringing the mixture to a boil. Once boiling, reduce the heat to low and let it simmer, uncovered, for about 20-25 minutes until the lentils are soft and have absorbed most of the liquid.
5. **Add Coconut Milk**: If using coconut milk, stir it in during the last 5 minutes of cooking. This adds a creamy texture and rich flavor to the dhal.
6. **Season and Adjust**: Taste the dhal and adjust the seasoning with salt and pepper as needed. If the mixture is too thick, you can add a splash more broth or water to reach your desired consistency.
7. **Serve and Garnish:** Remove from heat and ladle the *Red Lentil Dhal* into bowls. Garnish with fresh cilantro and serve with lime wedges on the side for an extra burst of flavor.

Nutritional Value (per serving, approximately 1 cup)

- **Calories**: ~220
- **Protein**: 12g
- **Carbohydrates**: 36g
- **Fiber**: 10g
- **Fat**: 6g
- **Saturated Fat**: 4g

- **Sugar**: 2g
- **Sodium**: 300mg
- **Potassium**: 550mg
- **Vitamin A**: 15% of daily recommended intake
- **Vitamin C**: 5% of daily recommended intake
- **Calcium**: 6% of daily recommended intake
- **Iron**: 20% of daily recommended intake

Red Lentil Dhal with Turmeric and Ginger is not only a delicious and comforting dish but also a powerhouse of nutrition. Packed with plant-based protein and fiber, it provides sustained energy and promotes digestive health. The use of turmeric and ginger adds a host of health benefits, including anti-inflammatory properties and digestive support, making this dhal a nutritious choice for everyone. Easy to prepare and adaptable to various dietary needs, this recipe can easily be customized with additional vegetables or spices according to your taste preferences. Enjoy this dish as a main course, paired with rice or naan, or as a hearty side alongside your favorite proteins. With its vibrant flavors and nutritional benefits, *Red Lentil Dhal* is sure to become a beloved staple in your culinary repertoire!

Zucchini and Basil Soup is a light, refreshing, and flavorful dish that perfectly showcases the delicate taste of zucchini combined with the aromatic essence of fresh basil. This vibrant green soup is not only visually appealing but also packed with nutrients, making it an ideal choice for a healthy appetizer or a light meal. Zucchini is low in calories and high in fiber, which helps to keep you feeling full while supporting digestive health. Basil adds a fragrant herbal note that elevates the soup's flavor profile, making each spoonful a delightful experience. This recipe is simple to prepare and can be made in just a matter of minutes, making it perfect for busy weeknights or when you want a quick, wholesome meal. For added creaminess, a splash of coconut milk or a dollop of Greek yogurt can be included, creating a silky texture that enhances the soup's richness. Enjoy *Zucchini and Basil Soup* warm or chilled, garnished with fresh basil leaves or a sprinkle of pine nuts for a delightful touch.

Preparation Time

- **Prep Time**: 10 minutes
- **Cook Time**: 20 minutes
- **Total Time**: 30 minutes

Ingredients

- 2 tablespoons olive oil
- 1 medium onion, chopped
- 2 cloves garlic, minced
- 4 medium zucchinis, chopped
- 4 cups vegetable broth
- 1 cup fresh basil leaves, packed
- 1 tablespoon lemon juice
- Salt and pepper to taste
- Optional garnish: Fresh basil leaves, croutons, or a swirl of coconut milk

Procedure

1. **Sauté the Onion and Garlic**: In a large pot, heat the olive oil over medium heat. Add the chopped onion and sauté for about 5 minutes until it becomes translucent. Stir in the minced garlic and cook for another minute until fragrant.

2. **Add Zucchini**: Add the chopped zucchini to the pot, stirring to combine with the onion and garlic. Cook for about 5 minutes until the zucchini begins to soften.

3. **Pour in Broth**: Pour in the vegetable broth, bringing the mixture to a boil. Once boiling, reduce the heat to low and let it simmer for about 10-15 minutes, or until the zucchini is fully tender.

4. **Blend the Soup**: Remove the pot from heat and add the fresh basil leaves to the soup. Using an immersion blender or a countertop blender, puree the soup until smooth. Be careful when blending hot liquids; you may need to allow it to cool slightly.

5. **Add Lemon Juice**: Once blended, return the soup to the pot (if using a countertop blender) and stir in the lemon juice. This adds brightness to the flavor.

6. **Season**: Taste the soup and season with salt and pepper to your liking. If the soup is too thick, you can add a bit more broth or water to reach your desired consistency.

7. **Serve and Garnish**: Ladle the *Zucchini and Basil Soup* into bowls. Garnish with fresh basil leaves, croutons, or a swirl of coconut milk, if desired. Serve warm or chilled, and enjoy!

Nutritional Value (per serving, approximately 1 cup)

- **Calories**: ~90
- **Protein**: 3g
- **Carbohydrates**: 13g
- **Fiber**: 3g
- **Fat**: 4g
- **Saturated Fat**: 0.5g
- **Sugar**: 3g
- **Sodium**: 250mg
- **Potassium**: 400mg
- **Vitamin A**: 10% of daily recommended intake

- **Vitamin C**: 25% of daily recommended intake
- **Calcium**: 4% of daily recommended intake
- **Iron**: 6% of daily recommended intake

Zucchini and Basil Soup is a delightful, healthful dish that offers a burst of flavor while being light on the palate. Packed with vitamins and minerals, this soup supports overall health and wellness, making it a perfect addition to your diet. The ease of preparation allows for a quick meal solution without sacrificing taste or nutrition. Feel free to customize the recipe by adding other vegetables or herbs according to your preferences. With its creamy texture and aromatic taste, this soup is sure to become a favorite for both casual dinners and special occasions. Enjoy the refreshing flavors of *Zucchini and Basil Soup* as a soothing and nourishing option that can be enjoyed any time of the year!

Chapter 5

Wholesome Main Courses

Salmon with Turmeric and Ginger Marinade is a vibrant and flavorful dish that combines the rich, buttery taste of salmon with the warm, earthy notes of turmeric and the zesty kick of ginger. This marinade not only infuses the fish with delightful flavors but also offers numerous health benefits due to the anti-inflammatory properties of both turmeric and ginger. Salmon is an excellent source of omega-3 fatty acids, which are known for their heart-healthy benefits and ability to reduce inflammation in the body. This recipe is quick to prepare, making it perfect for a weeknight dinner or a special occasion. The marinated salmon can be grilled, baked, or pan-seared, allowing for versatility in cooking methods. Paired with a side of steamed vegetables or a fresh salad, this dish becomes a nutritious meal that is both satisfying and nourishing. Enjoy the delicious flavors of this dish while reaping its health benefits!

Preparation Time

- **Prep Time**: 15 minutes
- **Cook Time**: 15 minutes
- **Total Time**: 30 minutes

Ingredients

- 4 salmon fillets (about 6 oz each)
- 2 tablespoons fresh ginger, grated
- 2 tablespoons turmeric powder
- 3 tablespoons soy sauce or tamari (for gluten-free option)
- 2 tablespoons honey or maple syrup
- 2 tablespoons olive oil
- Juice of 1 lime
- 2 cloves garlic, minced
- Salt and pepper to taste

- Fresh cilantro for garnish

Procedure

1. **Prepare the Marinade**: In a mixing bowl, combine the grated ginger, turmeric powder, soy sauce (or tamari), honey (or maple syrup), olive oil, lime juice, and minced garlic. Whisk until the ingredients are well blended and form a smooth marinade.

2. **Marinate the Salmon**: Place the salmon fillets in a shallow dish or a resealable plastic bag. Pour the marinade over the salmon, ensuring that each fillet is well coated. Cover the dish or seal the bag and let it marinate in the refrigerator for at least 15 minutes, or up to 1 hour for more intense flavor.

3. **Preheat the Cooking Surface**: If grilling, preheat the grill to medium-high heat. If baking, preheat the oven to 400°F (200°C). If pan-searing, heat a non-stick skillet over medium heat and add a little oil to prevent sticking.

4. **Cook the Salmon**: Remove the salmon from the marinade, allowing any excess marinade to drip off. Season with salt and pepper to taste. Cook the salmon for about 4-5 minutes on each side if grilling or pan-searing, or bake for 12-15 minutes in the oven, or until the fish is cooked through and flakes easily with a fork.

5. **Baste (Optional)**: If desired, during the last few minutes of cooking, brush the salmon with any remaining marinade for added flavor and moisture.

6. **Check for Doneness**: The internal temperature of the salmon should reach 145°F (63°C) for safe consumption. The fish should be opaque and easily flake with a fork.

7. **Serve and Garnish**: Once cooked, remove the salmon from the heat and let it rest for a minute. Serve the salmon garnished with fresh cilantro and lime wedges for an extra burst of flavor. Pair with your favorite sides, such as steamed vegetables or a quinoa salad.

Nutritional Value (per serving, approximately 6 oz)

- **Calories**: ~350
- **Protein**: 34g
- **Carbohydrates**: 12g
- **Fiber**: 1g

- **Fat**: 20g
- **Saturated Fat**: 3g
- **Sugar**: 6g
- **Sodium**: 600mg
- **Potassium**: 700mg
- **Vitamin A**: 10% of daily recommended intake
- **Vitamin C**: 15% of daily recommended intake
- **Calcium**: 2% of daily recommended intake
- **Iron**: 5% of daily recommended intake

Salmon with Turmeric and Ginger Marinade is not only delicious but also incredibly nutritious, making it a perfect addition to any meal plan focused on health and wellness. This dish is rich in protein and healthy fats, making it satisfying while supporting muscle health and overall well-being. The vibrant colors and bold flavors of the marinade create an appetizing presentation that is sure to impress family and guests alike. Feel free to customize the marinade by adding other herbs or spices to suit your taste. Enjoy this delectable salmon dish that is both easy to prepare and a treat for your taste buds!

Grilled Chicken with Avocado Salsa is a fresh, flavorful dish that perfectly combines the juicy tenderness of grilled chicken with a vibrant and zesty avocado salsa. This meal is ideal for warm weather dining, providing a light yet satisfying option that is both nutritious and delicious. The grilled chicken is seasoned to perfection, ensuring a rich flavor that pairs wonderfully with the creamy avocado, tangy lime juice, and refreshing cilantro in the salsa. This dish not only highlights the deliciousness of the ingredients but also offers a wealth of nutrients, including lean protein from the chicken and healthy fats from the avocado. It's a simple yet elegant recipe that can be prepared in a short amount of time, making it a great option for busy weeknights or weekend gatherings. Serve it with a side of brown rice, quinoa, or a fresh green salad for a complete meal. Enjoy this delightful dish that embodies the essence of healthy eating!

Preparation Time

- **Prep Time**: 15 minutes
- **Cook Time**: 15 minutes
- **Total Time**: 30 minutes

Ingredients

- **For the Chicken:**
  - 4 boneless, skinless chicken breasts (about 6 oz each)
  - 2 tablespoons olive oil
  - 1 teaspoon garlic powder
  - 1 teaspoon onion powder
  - 1 teaspoon smoked paprika
  - Salt and pepper to taste
  -

- **For the Avocado Salsa:**
  - 2 ripe avocados, diced
  - 1 medium tomato, diced
  - 1/4 cup red onion, finely chopped
  - 1 jalapeño, seeded and minced (optional)

  o 1/4 cup fresh cilantro, chopped

  o Juice of 2 limes

  o Salt to taste

Procedure

1. **Prepare the Chicken Marinade**: In a small bowl, mix together the olive oil, garlic powder, onion powder, smoked paprika, salt, and pepper. Coat the chicken breasts with this mixture, ensuring they are evenly seasoned. Allow the chicken to marinate for at least 10 minutes to enhance the flavor.

2. **Preheat the Grill**: Preheat your grill to medium-high heat. Make sure the grill grates are clean and lightly oiled to prevent sticking.

3. **Make the Avocado Salsa**: While the grill heats up, prepare the avocado salsa. In a medium bowl, combine the diced avocados, tomato, red onion, jalapeño (if using), cilantro, lime juice, and salt. Gently toss to combine, being careful not to mash the avocado. Set aside.

4. **Grill the Chicken**: Once the grill is hot, place the marinated chicken breasts on the grill. Cook for about 6-7 minutes on each side or until the chicken is cooked through and has nice grill marks. The internal temperature should reach 165°F (75°C).

5. **Rest the Chicken**: After grilling, remove the chicken from the grill and let it rest for about 5 minutes. This allows the juices to redistribute, ensuring tender and juicy chicken.

6. **Serve the Dish**: Slice the grilled chicken and place it on a serving platter or individual plates. Top each piece of chicken generously with the avocado salsa.

7. **Garnish and Enjoy**: Optionally, garnish with additional cilantro and lime wedges for a pop of color and flavor. Serve immediately with your choice of side dishes, such as brown rice or a green salad, and enjoy your delicious meal!

Nutritional Value (per serving, approximately 1 chicken breast with salsa)

- **Calories**: ~360
- **Protein**: 30g
- **Carbohydrates**: 14g
- **Fiber**: 7g

- **Fat**: 22g

- **Saturated Fat**: 3g

- **Sugar**: 2g

- **Sodium**: 350mg

- **Potassium**: 800mg

- **Vitamin A**: 8% of daily recommended intake

- **Vitamin C**: 25% of daily recommended intake

- **Calcium**: 4% of daily recommended intake

- **Iron**: 8% of daily recommended intake

Grilled Chicken with Avocado Salsa is not only a feast for the taste buds but also a well-rounded meal that supports overall health and wellness. The combination of lean protein from the chicken and healthy fats from the avocado makes this dish satisfying and nutritious. With its bright flavors and beautiful presentation, it's a fantastic option for summer barbecues, family dinners, or any occasion where you want to impress your guests. Enjoy this dish as part of your journey towards a healthier lifestyle while savoring every delicious bite!

Imagine a warm evening with friends gathered around the table, sharing stories and laughter. In the middle of the table, there's a vibrant platter of *Roasted Cauliflower Tacos with Spicy Yogurt Sauce*—a plant-based dish that not only looks colorful but is packed with layers of flavor. The crispy roasted cauliflower, seasoned with bold spices, pairs beautifully with the creamy and tangy yogurt sauce, which has just the right kick of heat. These tacos are the perfect blend of hearty, crunchy, and fresh, making them an ideal choice for anyone looking to enjoy a satisfying yet nutritious meal. Whether you're cooking for a weeknight family dinner or serving up something special for guests, this recipe is sure to be a crowd-pleaser.

Preparation Time

- **Prep Time**: 15 minutes
- **Cook Time**: 25 minutes
- **Total Time**: 40 minutes

Ingredients

For the Roasted Cauliflower:

- 1 large head of cauliflower, cut into small florets
- 2 tablespoons olive oil
- 1 teaspoon smoked paprika
- 1 teaspoon ground cumin
- 1/2 teaspoon garlic powder
- 1/2 teaspoon chili powder
- Salt and pepper to taste

For the Spicy Yogurt Sauce:

- 1 cup plain Greek yogurt
- 1 tablespoon hot sauce (adjust to taste)
- 1 teaspoon lime juice

- 1 clove garlic, minced
- Salt to taste

For the Tacos:

- 8 small corn or flour tortillas
- 1/4 cup fresh cilantro, chopped
- 1/4 red onion, finely chopped
- 1 avocado, sliced
- Lime wedges for serving

Procedure

1. **Preheat the Oven**: Begin by preheating your oven to 425°F (220°C). While the oven heats, prepare the cauliflower by cutting it into bite-sized florets. This step ensures that the cauliflower will roast evenly, becoming golden and crispy.
2. **Season the Cauliflower**: In a large bowl, toss the cauliflower florets with olive oil, smoked paprika, cumin, garlic powder, chili powder, salt, and pepper. Ensure the florets are evenly coated with the spices to bring out their flavor during roasting.
3. **Roast the Cauliflower**: Spread the seasoned cauliflower in a single layer on a baking sheet lined with parchment paper. Roast for 20-25 minutes, stirring halfway through, until the cauliflower is golden brown and crispy on the edges. This will give the tacos a satisfying crunch and deep, smoky flavor.
4. **Prepare the Spicy Yogurt Sauce**: While the cauliflower roasts, mix the yogurt, hot sauce, lime juice, minced garlic, and salt in a small bowl. Adjust the hot sauce according to your spice preference. The sauce should have a creamy, tangy base with a spicy kick that complements the roasted cauliflower.
5. **Warm the Tortillas**: Just before the cauliflower is ready, warm the tortillas either on a skillet or directly over a gas flame for a few seconds on each side until they're soft and pliable. This helps them hold the filling without tearing and adds a slight charred flavor.
6. **Assemble the Tacos**: Once the cauliflower is done roasting, start assembling the tacos. Place a few spoonfuls of roasted cauliflower onto each tortilla. Top with sliced avocado, chopped red onion, cilantro, and a generous drizzle of the spicy yogurt sauce.

7. **Serve and Enjoy**: Serve the tacos immediately, garnished with lime wedges for an extra burst of citrus flavor. You can also add any additional toppings like shredded lettuce or pickled jalapeños for more texture and spice. Enjoy these tacos with friends or family, knowing that you're treating them to a meal that's as wholesome as it is flavorful.

Nutritional Value (per serving, 2 tacos)

- **Calories**: ~300
- **Protein**: 10g
- **Carbohydrates**: 35g
- **Fiber**: 8g
- **Fat**: 15g
- **Saturated Fat**: 3g
- **Sugar**: 6g
- **Sodium**: 450mg
- **Potassium**: 700mg
- **Vitamin A**: 15% of daily recommended intake
- **Vitamin C**: 80% of daily recommended intake
- **Calcium**: 15% of daily recommended intake
- **Iron**: 10% of daily recommended intake

Roasted Cauliflower Tacos with Spicy Yogurt Sauce offer a delightful balance of textures and flavors. The cauliflower, with its crispy, smoky exterior, paired with the creamy avocado and fresh herbs, creates a taco experience that feels both indulgent and healthy. The yogurt sauce adds a spicy, tangy punch, cutting through the richness of the avocado and making each bite more exciting than the last. Best of all, this meal is plant-based, loaded with fiber, vitamins, and antioxidants, making it a perfect choice for those seeking a nutritious, anti-inflammatory diet.

Baked Cod with Lemon, Garlic & Olive Oil is a light and flavorful dish that showcases the delicate texture of fresh cod, perfectly balanced by the zesty brightness of lemon and the savory richness of garlic and olive oil. This Mediterranean-inspired recipe is simple to prepare yet impressively elegant, making it an excellent choice for both weeknight meals and special occasions. Cod, a lean and flaky white fish, is known for its mild flavor, making it an ideal canvas for bold seasonings like garlic and lemon. The gentle baking process ensures the fish remains moist and tender, while the olive oil adds heart-healthy fats and a smooth richness to the dish. Serve this baked cod alongside roasted vegetables or a fresh salad, and enjoy a wholesome meal that's not only delicious but packed with nutrients.

Preparation Time

- **Prep Time**: 10 minutes
- **Cook Time**: 15 minutes
- **Total Time**: 25 minutes

Ingredients

- 4 fresh cod fillets (about 6 oz each)
- 3 tablespoons extra virgin olive oil
- 3 cloves garlic, minced
- 1 large lemon (zested and juiced)
- 1 teaspoon dried oregano
- Salt and pepper to taste
- Fresh parsley, chopped (for garnish)
- Lemon wedges (for serving)

Procedure

1. **Preheat the Oven**: Preheat your oven to 400°F (200°C) and lightly grease a baking dish or line it with parchment paper to prevent sticking. The preheating ensures that the cod cooks evenly, preserving its tender texture.

2. **Prepare the Garlic Lemon Mixture**: In a small bowl, mix the olive oil, minced garlic, lemon zest, lemon juice, and dried oregano. This combination will serve as the flavorful marinade for the cod, infusing it with bright, zesty notes from the lemon and the aromatic essence of garlic.

3. **Season the Cod Fillets**: Arrange the cod fillets in the prepared baking dish in a single layer. Generously drizzle the lemon garlic mixture over each fillet, making sure to coat them evenly. Season with salt and pepper to taste. Allow the cod to sit for 5-10 minutes to absorb the flavors.

4. **Bake the Cod**: Place the baking dish in the preheated oven and bake for 12-15 minutes, or until the cod is opaque and flakes easily with a fork. Be careful not to overcook the fish to maintain its delicate texture.

5. **Check for Doneness**: Once the cod is baked, check the internal temperature with a meat thermometer—it should reach 145°F (63°C) when fully cooked. Alternatively, you can test by gently pressing the fillet; it should flake apart effortlessly.

6. **Garnish and Serve**: After removing the baked cod from the oven, sprinkle it with freshly chopped parsley for a burst of color and freshness. Serve each fillet with lemon wedges on the side for those who like an extra squeeze of citrus.

7. **Pair and Enjoy**: Pair the baked cod with a side of roasted vegetables, quinoa, or a simple green salad for a complete, nutritious meal. The subtle flavors of the fish will complement a wide variety of sides, and the light, bright dressing makes this dish feel indulgent yet healthy.

Nutritional Value (per serving, approximately 1 fillet)

- **Calories**: ~250
- **Protein**: 30g
- **Carbohydrates**: 2g

- **Fiber**: 0g
- **Fat**: 12g
- **Saturated Fat**: 2g
- **Cholesterol**: 60mg
- **Sodium**: 150mg
- **Potassium**: 650mg
- **Vitamin C**: 15% of daily recommended intake
- **Calcium**: 4% of daily recommended intake
- **Iron**: 6% of daily recommended intake

Baked Cod with Lemon, Garlic & Olive Oil is a simple yet flavorful dish that brings the natural taste of cod to life with minimal effort. The combination of lemon and garlic enhances the fish's mild flavor without overpowering it, while the olive oil ensures a moist, flaky texture. Rich in lean protein and low in calories, cod is an excellent source of essential nutrients such as potassium and B vitamins. Paired with heart-healthy fats from the olive oil and the antioxidant power of garlic and lemon, this dish is not only delicious but also promotes overall wellness. Whether you're cooking for yourself or entertaining guests, this recipe is a go-to for a quick, healthy, and flavorful meal.

Quinoa-Stuffed Bell Peppers is a vibrant, hearty, and nutritious dish that combines the richness of plant-based ingredients with the bold, fresh flavors of Mediterranean-inspired herbs and spices. The bell peppers, roasted to tender perfection, are filled with a delicious mixture of quinoa, vegetables, and flavorful seasonings, making this dish both satisfying and wholesome. Quinoa, a nutrient-dense grain, serves as a fantastic protein-packed base, while the bell peppers add a slightly sweet flavor and a crisp texture. This dish is perfect for a filling lunch or a light dinner and is an excellent option for meal prep as it reheats well. Whether you're serving it as a main course or a side, *Quinoa-Stuffed Bell Peppers* is a delightful way to incorporate anti-inflammatory ingredients into your diet.

Preparation Time

- **Prep Time**: 20 minutes
- **Cook Time**: 35 minutes
- **Total Time**: 55 minutes

Ingredients

- 4 large bell peppers (red, yellow, orange, or green)
- 1 cup quinoa, rinsed
- 2 cups vegetable broth (or water)
- 1 small onion, diced
- 2 cloves garlic, minced
- 1 cup diced tomatoes (fresh or canned)
- 1/2 cup black beans, drained and rinsed
- 1/2 cup corn kernels (fresh or frozen)
- 1 teaspoon cumin
- 1 teaspoon smoked paprika
- Salt and pepper to taste
- 2 tablespoons olive oil
- Fresh cilantro or parsley for garnish
- Lemon wedges for serving

Procedure

1. **Prepare the Quinoa**: Begin by rinsing the quinoa under cold water to remove its natural bitterness. Bring 2 cups of vegetable broth or water to a boil in a medium saucepan, then add the quinoa. Lower the heat to a simmer, cover, and cook for 15 minutes, or until the liquid is absorbed and the quinoa is fluffy. Fluff the quinoa with a fork and set it aside.

2. **Prepare the Bell Peppers**: While the quinoa cooks, preheat your oven to 375°F (190°C). Cut the tops off the bell peppers and remove the seeds and membranes inside. Lightly brush the peppers with olive oil and place them in a baking dish. Roast the bell peppers for 10 minutes, just until they start to soften, then remove them from the oven.

3. **Sauté the Vegetables**: In a large skillet, heat 1 tablespoon of olive oil over medium heat. Add the diced onion and sauté for 3-4 minutes until it becomes translucent. Add the minced garlic, cumin, and smoked paprika, stirring for another minute to release the aromatics. Stir in the diced tomatoes, black beans, and corn, and cook for an additional 5 minutes. Season with salt and pepper.

4. **Mix the Filling**: Once the vegetable mixture is cooked, combine it with the cooked quinoa in a large bowl. Stir well to ensure the ingredients are evenly distributed. Taste and adjust the seasoning if necessary. The quinoa and vegetable filling should be flavorful and well-spiced.

5. **Stuff the Peppers**: Generously stuff each bell pepper with the quinoa mixture, pressing it down gently to pack the filling inside. If you have extra filling, you can serve it on the side or use it in other meals. Drizzle the stuffed peppers with a little olive oil for added richness.

6. **Bake the Peppers**: Return the stuffed bell peppers to the oven and bake for 20-25 minutes, or until the peppers are tender and the filling is heated through. You can cover the dish with aluminum foil for the first 10 minutes to prevent the tops from browning too quickly.

7. **Garnish and Serve**: Once the stuffed peppers are done baking, remove them from the oven and garnish with freshly chopped cilantro or parsley. Serve the peppers with lemon wedges for a refreshing citrusy finish. These peppers are delicious on their own or paired with a simple green salad.

Nutritional Value (per serving, approximately 1 stuffed pepper)

- **Calories**: ~280
- **Protein**: 8g
- **Carbohydrates**: 45g
- **Fiber**: 10g
- **Fat**: 8g
- **Saturated Fat**: 1g
- **Sodium**: 450mg
- **Potassium**: 750mg
- **Vitamin A**: 100% of daily recommended intake
- **Vitamin C**: 300% of daily recommended intake
- **Calcium**: 6% of daily recommended intake
- **Iron**: 20% of daily recommended intake

Quinoa-Stuffed Bell Peppers is a nutrient-packed meal that offers a balance of protein, fiber, and healthy carbohydrates. Quinoa provides a complete protein source, essential for plant-based diets, while the black beans and vegetables contribute additional fiber and antioxidants. Bell peppers are naturally high in vitamin C, supporting immune health and providing an anti-inflammatory boost. This recipe is also highly versatile; you can adjust the seasonings or add other vegetables like zucchini or spinach for more variety. The dish is not only satisfying but also an excellent way to incorporate a rainbow of vegetables into your diet, supporting both gut health and overall wellness.

Sweet Potato and Chickpea Curry is a warm, hearty, and nourishing dish filled with rich spices and wholesome ingredients. This vegan-friendly curry combines the natural sweetness of sweet potatoes with the earthy, nutty flavor of chickpeas, simmered in a fragrant, coconut-based sauce. The combination of anti-inflammatory spices like turmeric, ginger, and cumin not only imparts incredible flavor but also offers various health benefits, making this dish both satisfying and nourishing. Perfect for a cozy meal, this curry can be enjoyed with basmati rice, quinoa, or warm flatbreads. It is a versatile recipe that can easily be adapted with your favorite vegetables or extra protein, and it's ideal for batch cooking or meal prepping as the flavors deepen over time.

Preparation Time

- **Prep Time**: 15 minutes
- **Cook Time**: 35 minutes
- **Total Time**: 50 minutes

Ingredients

- 2 medium sweet potatoes, peeled and diced
- 1 can (15 oz) chickpeas, drained and rinsed
- 1 tablespoon coconut oil
- 1 large onion, finely chopped
- 2 cloves garlic, minced
- 1 tablespoon fresh ginger, minced
- 1 tablespoon curry powder
- 1 teaspoon ground cumin
- 1 teaspoon ground turmeric
- 1 teaspoon ground coriander
- 1/2 teaspoon cayenne pepper (optional for heat)
- 1 can (14 oz) coconut milk
- 1 cup vegetable broth
- 1 can (14 oz) diced tomatoes
- Salt and pepper to taste

- Fresh cilantro, chopped (for garnish)
- Juice of 1 lime (for serving)

Procedure

1. **Sauté the Aromatics**: Heat the coconut oil in a large pot or Dutch oven over medium heat. Add the chopped onion and sauté for about 3-4 minutes until softened and translucent. Then, add the minced garlic and ginger, cooking for an additional 1-2 minutes until fragrant. These aromatics lay the foundation for the curry, bringing depth and richness to the dish.

2. **Add the Spices**: Stir in the curry powder, cumin, turmeric, ground coriander, and cayenne pepper (if using). Cook the spices for about 1 minute, stirring constantly, to toast them slightly and release their full flavor. Toasting the spices helps intensify their flavor, creating a more robust curry.

3. **Add the Sweet Potatoes and Chickpeas**: Add the diced sweet potatoes and chickpeas to the pot, stirring to coat them well with the aromatic spice mixture. Let them cook for about 2 minutes, absorbing the flavors. This ensures that every piece is seasoned before the liquid is added.

4. **Add the Liquids**: Pour in the coconut milk, vegetable broth, and diced tomatoes. Stir everything together, ensuring that the sweet potatoes and chickpeas are submerged in the liquid. Season with salt and pepper to taste. Bring the mixture to a gentle boil, then reduce the heat to low, allowing the curry to simmer.

5. **Simmer the Curry**: Cover the pot and let the curry simmer for 25-30 minutes, stirring occasionally. The sweet potatoes should become tender, and the sauce will thicken as it reduces. If you prefer a thicker consistency, remove the lid during the last 10 minutes of cooking.

6. **Check for Doneness**: Once the sweet potatoes are fully cooked and tender (they should easily be pierced with a fork), taste the curry and adjust the seasoning if needed. Add more salt, pepper, or additional cayenne for heat if desired. The sauce should be rich and flavorful, with a slight sweetness from the coconut milk and sweet potatoes.

7. **Garnish and Serve**: Remove the curry from the heat and stir in freshly chopped cilantro. Squeeze fresh lime juice over the top just before serving for a burst of brightness. Serve the curry over rice or with flatbreads, and enjoy the warm, comforting flavors.

Nutritional Value (per serving, approximately 1 cup of curry)

- **Calories**: ~320
- **Protein**: 8g
- **Carbohydrates**: 46g
- **Fiber**: 9g
- **Fat**: 12g
- **Saturated Fat**: 8g
- **Sodium**: 600mg
- **Potassium**: 800mg
- **Vitamin A**: 370% of daily recommended intake
- **Vitamin C**: 35% of daily recommended intake
- **Calcium**: 10% of daily recommended intake
- **Iron**: 20% of daily recommended intake

Sweet Potato and Chickpea Curry is a nutrient-dense meal that offers a balance of protein, fiber, and healthy fats. Sweet potatoes are packed with beta-carotene (vitamin A), which supports eye health and immune function, while chickpeas provide plant-based protein and fiber, aiding in digestion and satiety. The coconut milk adds a rich, creamy texture without the need for dairy, while the spices like turmeric and ginger contribute anti-inflammatory properties. This curry is not only delicious but also supports overall health and wellness with its blend of vitamins, minerals, and anti-inflammatory ingredients.

Sautéed Tempeh with Ginger and Sesame is a flavorful, protein-rich dish that highlights the nutty taste and hearty texture of tempeh. This plant-based protein is sautéed to golden perfection and infused with the fresh flavors of ginger, garlic, sesame oil, and tamari (soy sauce). Ginger adds a zesty, anti-inflammatory boost while the sesame oil and seeds lend a rich, nutty depth to the dish. This recipe is simple yet packed with umami and can be served as a standalone dish, over a bed of rice, or as part of a larger meal. It's a versatile, healthy option for anyone looking to incorporate more plant-based proteins and anti-inflammatory ingredients into their diet.

Preparation Time

- **Prep Time**: 10 minutes
- **Cook Time**: 15 minutes
- **Total Time**: 25 minutes

Ingredients

- 1 (8 oz) package of tempeh, sliced into thin strips or cubes
- 1 tablespoon sesame oil
- 2 cloves garlic, minced
- 1 tablespoon fresh ginger, minced
- 2 tablespoons tamari (or low-sodium soy sauce)
- 1 tablespoon rice vinegar
- 1 tablespoon maple syrup or honey (optional for a touch of sweetness)
- 1 tablespoon sesame seeds, toasted
- 2 green onions, sliced (for garnish)
- 1/4 teaspoon crushed red pepper flakes (optional for heat)
- Steamed rice or quinoa (for serving)

Procedure

1. **Prepare the Tempeh**: Begin by slicing the tempeh into thin strips or small cubes, depending on your preference. If you want to remove some of the tempeh's slightly bitter taste, you can steam it for 5 minutes before sautéing, but this step is optional. Steaming helps to soften the tempeh and allows it to absorb flavors more readily.

2. **Heat the Oil**: In a large skillet or wok, heat the sesame oil over medium heat. Sesame oil has a low smoke point, so ensure the heat is moderate to prevent burning. Once the oil is shimmering, add the tempeh slices in a single layer and sauté them for 3-4 minutes on each side, until golden brown and slightly crispy.

3. **Add the Aromatics**: Once the tempeh is golden, reduce the heat to low and add the minced garlic and ginger to the skillet. Sauté the aromatics for about 1 minute, stirring constantly to prevent them from burning. The garlic and ginger should become fragrant and infuse the tempeh with their rich flavors.

4. **Add the Sauce**: Pour in the tamari, rice vinegar, and maple syrup (if using). Stir well to coat the tempeh evenly with the sauce. The combination of tamari and vinegar will provide a savory and slightly tangy balance, while the maple syrup adds a subtle sweetness to complement the dish.

5. **Simmer to Glaze**: Allow the sauce to simmer for 2-3 minutes, letting it reduce and thicken slightly. Stir occasionally to ensure the tempeh is evenly coated. As the sauce reduces, it will form a delicious glaze on the tempeh, locking in the flavor.

6. **Add the Sesame Seeds**: Once the sauce has thickened, sprinkle in the toasted sesame seeds and toss to combine. The sesame seeds add a lovely crunch and nutty flavor to the dish. At this point, you can also sprinkle crushed red pepper flakes for a bit of heat if desired.

7. **Garnish and Serve**: Remove the skillet from the heat and transfer the tempeh to a serving plate. Garnish with sliced green onions for a fresh burst of flavor. Serve the sautéed tempeh over steamed rice or quinoa for a complete, balanced meal, or as a topping for stir-fried vegetables.

Nutritional Value (per serving, approximately 1 cup of sautéed tempeh)

- **Calories**: ~250
- **Protein**: 18g
- **Carbohydrates**: 15g
- **Fiber**: 5g
- **Fat**: 12g
- **Saturated Fat**: 2g
- **Sodium**: 600mg
- **Iron**: 15% of daily recommended intake
- **Calcium**: 10% of daily recommended intake
- **Vitamin B12**: 20% of daily recommended intake (from tempeh)
- **Magnesium**: 25% of daily recommended intake

Sautéed Tempeh with Ginger and Sesame is a nutrient-dense dish that provides a substantial amount of plant-based protein, making it an excellent meat alternative for those following a vegetarian or vegan diet. Tempeh, made from fermented soybeans, is rich in probiotics, aiding digestion and gut health. It also contains essential vitamins and minerals such as calcium, iron, and magnesium, supporting bone health and immune function. The ginger and garlic not only contribute to the robust flavor but also offer powerful anti-inflammatory properties. This dish is perfect for those looking to incorporate wholesome, anti-inflammatory ingredients into a quick, satisfying meal.

Zucchini Noodles with Pesto and Cherry Tomatoes is a light, refreshing, and nutrient-packed dish that replaces traditional pasta with spiralized zucchini. Zucchini noodles, also known as "zoodles," offer a low-carb, gluten-free alternative to regular pasta, making this dish perfect for those looking for a healthy, quick meal. The vibrant green pesto adds a rich, savory flavor, while the burst of sweet cherry tomatoes balances the dish. This recipe is not only delicious but also packed with anti-inflammatory ingredients like fresh basil, garlic, and olive oil, making it a great choice for supporting overall wellness.

Preparation Time

- **Prep Time**: 10 minutes
- **Cook Time**: 5 minutes
- **Total Time**: 15 minutes

Ingredients

- 4 medium zucchinis, spiralized into noodles
- 1 cup fresh basil leaves
- 1/4 cup pine nuts or walnuts
- 1/3 cup extra virgin olive oil
- 2 cloves garlic, minced
- 1/4 cup nutritional yeast or grated Parmesan cheese (for a non-vegan option)
- Juice of 1 lemon
- Salt and pepper to taste
- 1 cup cherry tomatoes, halved
- 1 tablespoon olive oil (for sautéing the noodles)
- Crushed red pepper flakes (optional for heat)

Procedure

1. **Prepare the Pesto**: In a food processor, combine the fresh basil leaves, pine nuts (or walnuts), minced garlic, nutritional yeast (or Parmesan), lemon juice, and a pinch of salt and pepper. Pulse until the ingredients are finely chopped. Then, with the motor running, slowly drizzle in the olive oil until the pesto reaches a smooth consistency. Taste and adjust the seasoning, adding more salt, pepper, or lemon juice as needed. This vibrant green pesto is the heart of the dish, providing a rich, savory flavor.

2. **Spiralize the Zucchini**: Using a spiralizer, create long, thin noodles from the zucchinis. If you don't have a spiralizer, you can use a vegetable peeler to create ribbon-like strands. Zucchini noodles (or zoodles) are a fantastic low-carb, gluten-free alternative to traditional pasta, offering a fresh and light base for the dish.

3. **Sauté the Zoodles**: Heat 1 tablespoon of olive oil in a large skillet over medium heat. Add the zucchini noodles and sauté for about 2-3 minutes, tossing frequently, until they are just tender but still slightly firm (al dente). Be careful not to overcook the zoodles, as they can release too much moisture and become mushy.

4. **Add the Cherry Tomatoes**: Once the zoodles are tender, add the halved cherry tomatoes to the skillet. Sauté for an additional 1-2 minutes until the tomatoes are warmed through but still hold their shape. The sweet, juicy cherry tomatoes add a burst of color and flavor, balancing the savory pesto.

5. **Combine with Pesto**: Remove the skillet from the heat and toss the sautéed zucchini noodles and tomatoes with the prepared pesto sauce. Make sure the zoodles are evenly coated with the rich pesto, ensuring every bite is flavorful.

6. **Season and Serve**: Sprinkle the dish with a little more salt and pepper to taste. If you like a bit of heat, add a pinch of crushed red pepper flakes. This final touch adds a subtle kick, balancing the freshness of the zucchini and the brightness of the pesto.

7. **Garnish and Enjoy**: Serve the zucchini noodles in bowls, garnishing with extra fresh basil leaves and a sprinkle of nutritional yeast or Parmesan. Enjoy this light yet satisfying dish on its own or pair it with a simple side salad for a complete meal.

Nutritional Value (per serving, approximately 1 bowl)

- **Calories**: ~230
- **Protein**: 7g
- **Carbohydrates**: 11g
- **Fiber**: 4g
- **Fat**: 19g
- **Saturated Fat**: 2.5g
- **Sodium**: 150mg
- **Potassium**: 500mg
- **Vitamin C**: 50% of daily recommended intake
- **Vitamin A**: 25% of daily recommended intake
- **Calcium**: 10% of daily recommended intake
- **Iron**: 10% of daily recommended intake

Zucchini Noodles with Pesto and Cherry Tomatoes is a nutritious, low-calorie meal that's rich in healthy fats, fiber, and essential vitamins. Zucchini is high in water content and low in carbohydrates, making it a perfect base for a light meal. Basil, the star ingredient in pesto, contains potent anti-inflammatory compounds like eugenol, while garlic and olive oil are known for their heart-healthy benefits. Cherry tomatoes are packed with antioxidants like lycopene and vitamin C, supporting immune health and reducing inflammation. This dish is not only delicious but also an excellent option for those looking to enhance their diet with anti-inflammatory, plant-based ingredients.

CHAPTER 6

Side Dishes Packed With Flavor

Roasted Brussels Sprouts with Balsamic Glaze

Roasted Brussels Sprouts with Balsamic Glaze is a simple yet flavorful side dish that highlights the natural nuttiness and crispiness of roasted Brussels sprouts, enhanced by the rich, tangy sweetness of a balsamic glaze. Brussels sprouts, a cruciferous vegetable, are rich in vitamins and minerals and have potent anti-inflammatory properties. The roasting process brings out their natural sweetness, while the balsamic glaze adds a luscious, caramelized touch that balances the slightly bitter notes of the sprouts. This dish is perfect as a side for a main course or even as a snack for those looking to incorporate more vegetables into their diet.

Preparation Time

- **Prep Time**: 10 minutes
- **Cook Time**: 25 minutes
- **Total Time**: 35 minutes

Ingredients

- 1 ½ pounds Brussels sprouts, trimmed and halved
- 2 tablespoons extra virgin olive oil
- 1 tablespoon balsamic vinegar
- 1 tablespoon maple syrup (optional for added sweetness)
- Salt and pepper to taste
- 1/4 cup balsamic glaze (store-bought or homemade)
- 1 tablespoon toasted pine nuts (optional for garnish)
- Fresh thyme or parsley (optional for garnish)

Procedure

1. **Preheat the Oven**: Preheat your oven to 400°F (200°C). Line a large baking sheet with parchment paper or lightly grease it with olive oil to prevent sticking. Preheating the oven ensures that the Brussels sprouts will roast evenly and develop a crispy, caramelized exterior.

2. **Prepare the Brussels Sprouts**: Rinse and trim the Brussels sprouts, cutting off the tough ends and removing any damaged outer leaves. Cut each sprout in half lengthwise to ensure even cooking. Halving them also allows for maximum surface area contact with the heat, which helps create a crispy, golden-brown texture.

3. **Toss with Olive Oil and Seasoning**: Place the halved Brussels sprouts in a large bowl. Drizzle them with the extra virgin olive oil, balsamic vinegar, and optional maple syrup. Season with salt and pepper, and toss well to ensure all the sprouts are evenly coated. The balsamic and maple syrup combination creates a sweet-tangy balance that complements the roasted sprouts beautifully.

4. **Roast the Brussels Sprouts**: Spread the Brussels sprouts in a single layer on the prepared baking sheet, cut side down. Roast them in the preheated oven for 20-25 minutes, tossing once halfway through. The sprouts are done when they are golden brown and crispy on the outside, tender on the inside, and slightly caramelized.

5. **Prepare the Balsamic Glaze**: If you're using store-bought balsamic glaze, you can skip this step. If making your own, heat 1/2 cup of balsamic vinegar in a small saucepan over medium heat. Allow it to simmer and reduce by half, about 5-7 minutes, until thickened to a syrupy consistency. This glaze adds a rich, tangy sweetness to the dish that perfectly complements the savory sprouts.

6. **Drizzle the Balsamic Glaze**: Once the Brussels sprouts are roasted to perfection, remove them from the oven and transfer them to a serving dish. Drizzle the balsamic glaze generously over the top, ensuring each sprout gets a touch of that deliciously sweet and tangy flavor. You can add more or less glaze depending on your preference.

7. **Garnish and Serve**: For an extra layer of flavor and texture, garnish the roasted Brussels sprouts with toasted pine nuts and fresh herbs like thyme or parsley. Serve immediately as

a side dish or a healthy snack. The pine nuts add a nutty crunch, while the fresh herbs brighten up the dish.

Nutritional Value (per serving, approximately 1 cup)

- **Calories**: ~150
- **Protein**: 4g
- **Carbohydrates**: 15g
- **Fiber**: 5g
- **Fat**: 8g
- **Saturated Fat**: 1g
- **Sugar**: 6g (includes natural sugars from the maple syrup and balsamic glaze)
- **Sodium**: 150mg
- **Vitamin C**: 80% of daily recommended intake
- **Vitamin K**: 220% of daily recommended intake
- **Folate**: 10% of daily recommended intake
- **Potassium**: 10% of daily recommended intake

Roasted Brussels Sprouts with Balsamic Glaze is a nutrient-rich, anti-inflammatory dish that delivers an array of health benefits. Brussels sprouts are an excellent source of fiber, vitamins C and K, and antioxidants like sulforaphane, which helps reduce inflammation and supports detoxification in the body. The olive oil provides heart-healthy fats, while the balsamic vinegar adds a dose of polyphenols, known for their antioxidant and anti-inflammatory properties. This dish is not only delicious but also a fantastic way to incorporate more greens into your diet with minimal effort.

Turmeric-Spiced Sweet Potato Fries are a healthier, anti-inflammatory twist on classic fries. This recipe combines the natural sweetness of sweet potatoes with the earthy warmth of turmeric, making it both flavorful and nutritious. These fries are baked, not fried, which helps to retain their nutritional value while keeping them light and crispy. The addition of turmeric not only adds a bright golden hue but also provides anti-inflammatory benefits, thanks to the curcumin compound found in turmeric. These fries are perfect as a side dish, snack, or even as part of a wholesome bowl meal.

Preparation Time

- **Prep Time**: 10 minutes
- **Cook Time**: 25-30 minutes
- **Total Time**: 35-40 minutes

Ingredients

- 2 large sweet potatoes, peeled and cut into thin fries
- 2 tablespoons olive oil
- 1 teaspoon ground turmeric
- 1/2 teaspoon smoked paprika
- 1/2 teaspoon garlic powder
- 1/2 teaspoon ground cumin (optional)
- 1/4 teaspoon black pepper
- Salt to taste
- 1 tablespoon cornstarch (optional, for extra crispiness)
- Fresh parsley, chopped (optional, for garnish)

Procedure

1. **Preheat the Oven**: Preheat your oven to 425°F (220°C). Line a large baking sheet with parchment paper or lightly grease it with olive oil. Preheating the oven ensures the fries bake evenly and achieve a crispy texture.

2. **Prepare the Sweet Potatoes**: Peel and slice the sweet potatoes into even-sized thin fries, about 1/4-inch thick. Try to cut them as uniformly as possible to ensure that they bake evenly. The thinner the fries, the crispier they'll get in the oven.

3. **Season the Fries**: In a large mixing bowl, toss the sweet potato fries with olive oil, turmeric, smoked paprika, garlic powder, black pepper, and salt. Optionally, add ground cumin for a bit of extra warmth and depth. For extra crispiness, toss the fries in cornstarch before adding the oil and spices. This helps to create a light coating, resulting in a crunchier texture.

4. **Arrange on the Baking Sheet**: Spread the seasoned fries out in a single layer on the prepared baking sheet. Be careful not to overcrowd the pan, as this can lead to soggy fries. If necessary, use two baking sheets to ensure the fries have enough space to roast properly.

5. **Bake the Fries**: Place the baking sheet in the preheated oven and bake the fries for 25-30 minutes, flipping them halfway through. This ensures they cook evenly and get crispy on both sides. Watch them carefully in the last 5 minutes to prevent burning.

6. **Check for Doneness**: The fries are ready when they're golden brown and crispy on the edges, but still tender on the inside. If you prefer extra crispy fries, you can leave them in the oven for an additional 5 minutes. Once done, remove the fries from the oven and let them cool slightly before serving.

7. **Garnish and Serve**: Transfer the fries to a serving platter, sprinkle with fresh parsley for a pop of color, and serve with your favorite dipping sauce, such as a tangy yogurt-based dip or a spiced tahini sauce. Enjoy these flavorful, turmeric-infused sweet potato fries as a healthier alternative to traditional fries.

Nutritional Value (per serving, approximately 1 cup)

- **Calories**: ~180
- **Protein**: 2g
- **Carbohydrates**: 30g
- **Fiber**: 4g
- **Fat**: 7g
- **Saturated Fat**: 1g
- **Sugar**: 7g (naturally occurring from sweet potatoes)
- **Sodium**: 200mg

- **Vitamin A**: 370% of daily recommended intake
- **Vitamin C**: 15% of daily recommended intake
- **Potassium**: 12% of daily recommended intake
- **Iron**: 5% of daily recommended intake

Turmeric-Spiced Sweet Potato Fries are not only a tasty side dish but also packed with nutritional benefits. Sweet potatoes are rich in beta-carotene, which converts to vitamin A in the body, supporting eye health and immune function. Turmeric, known for its anti-inflammatory properties, helps reduce inflammation in the body, making these fries a great addition to any anti-inflammatory diet. The olive oil provides heart-healthy fats, while the spices like garlic powder and smoked paprika add depth without adding unnecessary calories. These fries are a guilt-free, delicious way to enjoy a comforting snack or side dish with an anti-inflammatory boost.

Ginger Garlic Green Beans are a quick, delicious, and nutrient-packed side dish that combines fresh green beans with the bold flavors of ginger and garlic. The vibrant green beans retain their crunch while absorbing the savory and slightly spicy notes from the ginger and garlic, making this dish a flavorful and anti-inflammatory powerhouse. It's perfect as a side for main meals or even as a light, healthy snack. Both ginger and garlic are known for their anti-inflammatory and immune-boosting properties, which make this dish as nutritious as it is tasty.

Preparation Time

- **Prep Time**: 10 minutes
- **Cook Time**: 10 minutes
- **Total Time**: 20 minutes

Ingredients

- 1 pound (about 450g) fresh green beans, trimmed
- 1 tablespoon olive oil or sesame oil
- 3 garlic cloves, minced
- 1 tablespoon fresh ginger, minced or grated
- 1 tablespoon low-sodium soy sauce (or tamari for gluten-free)
- 1 teaspoon rice vinegar (optional for a tangy kick)
- 1/2 teaspoon crushed red pepper flakes (optional for heat)
- Salt and pepper to taste
- 1 teaspoon sesame seeds (optional for garnish)

Procedure

1. **Blanch the Green Beans**: Start by bringing a large pot of salted water to a boil. Add the trimmed green beans to the pot and blanch them for 2-3 minutes, or until they turn bright green and are just tender but still crisp. Blanching the green beans first ensures that they retain their vibrant color and texture while reducing their cooking time in the pan.

2. **Shock the Green Beans**: Once the green beans are blanched, drain them immediately and transfer them to a bowl of ice water. This stops the cooking process and helps keep the beans crisp and vibrant. Let them sit in the ice water for about a minute before draining and setting them aside.

3. **Sauté the Garlic and Ginger**: In a large skillet or wok, heat 1 tablespoon of olive oil (or sesame oil for a nuttier flavor) over medium heat. Add the minced garlic and fresh ginger to the pan, sautéing for 1-2 minutes until fragrant and golden. Be careful not to burn the garlic, as it can become bitter.

4. **Add the Green Beans**: Once the garlic and ginger are cooked, add the drained green beans to the skillet. Toss the beans in the garlic and ginger mixture, coating them evenly with the oil and spices. Cook for 3-4 minutes, stirring frequently, until the green beans are heated through and slightly tender.

5. **Season with Soy Sauce**: Add the low-sodium soy sauce to the skillet, stirring to coat the green beans evenly. The soy sauce adds a savory umami flavor that complements the ginger and garlic. If desired, add a splash of rice vinegar for a hint of tanginess, and crushed red pepper flakes for a bit of heat. Cook for another 1-2 minutes, letting the sauce reduce slightly.

6. **Taste and Adjust**: Taste the green beans and adjust seasoning as needed. You can add more soy sauce for saltiness or a dash of black pepper to enhance the flavor. Remove the skillet from the heat once the beans are tender but still have a slight crunch.

7. **Serve and Garnish**: Transfer the Ginger Garlic Green Beans to a serving dish and sprinkle with sesame seeds for garnish if desired. Serve hot as a side dish with your favorite protein or grain, or enjoy them as a light, nutrient-rich snack.

Nutritional Value (per serving, approximately 1 cup)

- **Calories**: ~80
- **Protein**: 2g
- **Carbohydrates**: 10g
- **Fiber**: 4g
- **Fat**: 3g
- **Saturated Fat**: 0.5g

- **Sugar**: 3g (naturally occurring from green beans)
- **Sodium**: 180mg
- **Vitamin A**: 15% of daily recommended intake
- **Vitamin C**: 20% of daily recommended intake
- **Calcium**: 5% of daily recommended intake
- **Iron**: 6% of daily recommended intake

Ginger Garlic Green Beans are packed with nutrients and anti-inflammatory properties. Green beans are an excellent source of fiber, vitamins A and C, and antioxidants that support overall health and reduce inflammation. Ginger and garlic not only provide bold flavor but also offer immune-boosting and anti-inflammatory benefits. Ginger helps to ease digestion and reduce inflammation in the body, while garlic is known for its antiviral and antibacterial properties. The olive oil adds heart-healthy fats, making this dish both delicious and beneficial for a well-balanced, anti-inflammatory diet.

Roasted Beetroot with Thyme is a simple yet flavorful dish that highlights the natural sweetness of beets while infusing them with the earthy aroma of fresh thyme. Beets are rich in antioxidants, vitamins, and minerals, making this recipe not only delicious but also highly nutritious. Roasting the beets brings out their natural sweetness and enhances their deep, earthy flavor. This dish can be served as a side, added to salads, or paired with grains and proteins for a complete meal. The combination of beets and thyme is a perfect way to elevate a humble root vegetable into a flavorful and health-boosting meal.

Preparation Time

- **Prep Time**: 10 minutes
- **Cook Time**: 40-45 minutes
- **Total Time**: 50-55 minutes

Ingredients

- 4 medium beetroots, scrubbed and trimmed
- 2 tablespoons olive oil
- 1 tablespoon fresh thyme leaves (or 1 teaspoon dried thyme)
- 1 clove garlic, minced (optional for added flavor)
- Salt to taste
- Black pepper to taste
- 1 tablespoon balsamic vinegar (optional, for a tangy finish)

Procedure

1. **Preheat the Oven**: Preheat your oven to 400°F (200°C). Line a baking sheet with parchment paper or lightly grease it with olive oil. This ensures that the beets cook evenly and don't stick to the pan during roasting.

2. **Prepare the Beetroots**: Scrub the beetroots thoroughly to remove any dirt. Trim off the beet greens and the root ends. You can peel the beets if you prefer a smoother texture, but leaving the skin on can add extra nutrients and a rustic feel. Cut the beetroots into even-sized wedges or cubes, about 1-inch thick.

3. **Season the Beets**: Place the beetroot wedges in a large mixing bowl. Drizzle with olive oil and toss to coat evenly. Add the fresh thyme leaves, minced garlic (if using), and season generously with salt and pepper. Toss again to ensure that the beets are evenly coated with the seasonings and oil.

4. **Roast the Beets**: Spread the seasoned beetroot wedges in a single layer on the prepared baking sheet. Make sure they are not crowded, as this allows the heat to circulate and roast them evenly. Roast in the preheated oven for 40-45 minutes, turning them halfway through to ensure even cooking.

5. **Check for Doneness**: After 40-45 minutes, check the beets for tenderness by inserting a fork or knife into the thickest piece. The beets should be tender on the inside with slightly crispy, caramelized edges. If they need more time, roast for an additional 5-10 minutes, checking periodically to avoid overcooking.

6. **Add Balsamic Vinegar (Optional)**: If desired, remove the beets from the oven and drizzle with balsamic vinegar. This adds a tangy sweetness that complements the earthy flavor of the beets. Toss the beets lightly on the baking sheet to coat them with the vinegar.

7. **Serve**: Transfer the roasted beetroot to a serving dish. Garnish with a few extra fresh thyme leaves for added aroma and presentation. Serve hot or at room temperature as a side dish, or add to salads, grain bowls, or top with goat cheese for a complete, flavorful meal.

Nutritional Value (per serving, approximately 1 cup)

- **Calories**: ~110
- **Protein**: 2g
- **Carbohydrates**: 15g
- **Fiber**: 4g
- **Fat**: 5g
- **Saturated Fat**: 1g
- **Sugar**: 9g (naturally occurring from beets)
- **Sodium**: 200mg
- **Potassium**: 9% of daily recommended intake
- **Vitamin C**: 10% of daily recommended intake
- **Iron**: 6% of daily recommended intake

- **Folate**: 20% of daily recommended intake

Roasted Beetroot with Thyme is not only delicious but also packed with health benefits. Beetroots are an excellent source of dietary fiber, folate, and potassium. They are rich in antioxidants like betalains, which have anti-inflammatory and detoxifying properties. Thyme adds an earthy and aromatic note, while garlic provides an immune-boosting and anti-inflammatory benefit. Olive oil contributes healthy fats, which help the body absorb fat-soluble vitamins. This simple yet nutritious recipe is a great addition to an anti-inflammatory diet, supporting heart health, digestion, and overall well-being.

Quinoa Pilaf with Toasted Almonds and Cranberries

Quinoa Pilaf with Toasted Almonds and Cranberries is a hearty, nutritious dish that combines the nutty flavors of quinoa with the sweetness of dried cranberries and the crunch of toasted almonds. This recipe is a perfect side dish or light meal, offering a balance of protein, fiber, healthy fats, and antioxidants. Quinoa, a gluten-free ancient grain, is a complete protein, making it an excellent choice for plant-based diets. The addition of cranberries provides a sweet, tangy contrast to the savory quinoa, while almonds add texture and a boost of healthy fats. This dish is ideal for an anti-inflammatory diet and can be paired with roasted vegetables or proteins for a complete meal.

Preparation Time

- **Prep Time**: 10 minutes
- **Cook Time**: 20 minutes
- **Total Time**: 30 minutes

Ingredients

- 1 cup quinoa, rinsed
- 2 cups low-sodium vegetable broth (or water)
- 1/2 cup dried cranberries

- 1/3 cup sliced almonds, toasted
- 1 small onion, finely chopped
- 2 tablespoons olive oil
- 1 garlic clove, minced
- 1/2 teaspoon ground cumin
- Salt and pepper to taste
- 2 tablespoons fresh parsley, chopped (optional, for garnish)
- 1 tablespoon lemon juice (optional, for a zesty finish)

Procedure

1. **Toast the Almonds**: Begin by toasting the sliced almonds. Heat a small dry skillet over medium heat and add the almonds. Stir frequently for 3-5 minutes until they turn golden brown and fragrant. Be careful not to burn them. Once toasted, remove from the pan and set aside to cool. Toasting the almonds enhances their flavor and adds a delightful crunch to the dish.

2. **Sauté the Onion and Garlic**: In a medium saucepan, heat 2 tablespoons of olive oil over medium heat. Add the finely chopped onion and sauté for 3-4 minutes until softened and translucent. Then, add the minced garlic and ground cumin, stirring for about 1 minute until the garlic is fragrant and the cumin is well combined with the onion. This creates a savory base for the quinoa and infuses the dish with flavor.

3. **Cook the Quinoa**: Add the rinsed quinoa to the saucepan with the onion and garlic mixture, stirring to coat the quinoa with the oil and spices. Pour in the vegetable broth or water and bring the mixture to a boil. Once boiling, reduce the heat to low, cover the saucepan, and simmer for about 15 minutes, or until the quinoa has absorbed all the liquid and is tender. Fluff the quinoa with a fork to loosen the grains.

4. **Add the Cranberries**: Once the quinoa is fully cooked and fluffy, stir in the dried cranberries. The residual heat will soften the cranberries, allowing their natural sweetness to infuse the dish. This adds a touch of tart sweetness that balances the savory flavors of the pilaf.

5. **Mix in the Almonds**: Gently fold the toasted almonds into the quinoa and cranberry mixture. The crunchy texture of the almonds adds a delightful contrast to the soft quinoa and chewy cranberries. Make sure the almonds are evenly distributed throughout the dish.

6. **Season and Finish**: Season the quinoa pilaf with salt and pepper to taste. For an optional zesty finish, drizzle the dish with fresh lemon juice to brighten the flavors. The lemon juice will add a refreshing tang that complements the sweetness of the cranberries and the nuttiness of the quinoa.

7. **Garnish and Serve**: Transfer the quinoa pilaf to a serving dish and sprinkle with freshly chopped parsley for a burst of color and added freshness. Serve the pilaf warm as a side dish, or enjoy it as a light, nutrient-packed main course. It pairs well with roasted vegetables, grilled chicken, or fish.

Nutritional Value (per serving, approximately 1 cup)

- **Calories**: ~280
- **Protein**: 7g
- **Carbohydrates**: 34g
- **Fiber**: 5g
- **Fat**: 13g
- **Saturated Fat**: 1g
- **Sugar**: 8g (mostly from dried cranberries)
- **Sodium**: 150mg (varies with the use of broth or water)
- **Vitamin E**: 10% of daily recommended intake (from almonds)
- **Magnesium**: 20% of daily recommended intake (from quinoa and almonds)
- **Folate**: 10% of daily recommended intake
- **Iron**: 15% of daily recommended intake

Quinoa Pilaf with Toasted Almonds and Cranberries is a nutrient-dense dish that provides a complete source of plant-based protein, thanks to quinoa. It is rich in fiber, which supports digestion and helps regulate blood sugar levels. The almonds provide healthy fats, including vitamin E, which is beneficial for skin health and has anti-inflammatory properties. Cranberries are packed with antioxidants, particularly vitamin C, and contribute to reducing inflammation in the body. This dish is a delicious and nutritious addition to any anti-inflammatory diet, promoting overall health and well-being.

Grilled Asparagus with Lemon Zest

Grilled Asparagus with Lemon Zest is a simple yet elegant dish that highlights the natural flavors of fresh asparagus while adding a bright, citrusy note. Asparagus is a nutrient-rich vegetable packed with vitamins A, C, E, and K, as well as fiber and folate, making it an excellent choice for a healthy diet. Grilling enhances the asparagus' flavor, providing a delicious char while keeping the spears tender and crisp. The addition of lemon zest not only adds a refreshing zing but also elevates the dish, making it a perfect side for grilled meats, fish, or as part of a vibrant salad. This dish is quick to prepare and offers a delightful balance of flavors and textures.

Preparation Time

- **Prep Time**: 10 minutes
- **Cook Time**: 10 minutes
- **Total Time**: 20 minutes

Ingredients

- 1 pound fresh asparagus, trimmed
- 2 tablespoons olive oil
- Zest of 1 lemon
- 1 tablespoon fresh lemon juice
- Salt and pepper to taste
- 1 clove garlic, minced (optional for added flavor)
- 1 tablespoon grated Parmesan cheese (optional, for serving)
- Lemon wedges (for garnish)

Procedure

1. **Prepare the Asparagus**: Rinse the asparagus under cold water to remove any dirt or grit. Trim the tough ends of the asparagus spears, cutting off about 1-2 inches from the bottom. This will ensure that you have tender and edible pieces. Pat the asparagus dry with a clean kitchen towel or paper towel to remove excess moisture, which helps with grilling.

2. **Marinate the Asparagus**: In a large mixing bowl, combine the trimmed asparagus with olive oil, lemon zest, and lemon juice. If using garlic, add it to the mixture. Toss the asparagus gently to coat all the spears evenly with the marinade. Allow the asparagus to sit for about 5 minutes to absorb the flavors while you preheat the grill.

3. **Preheat the Grill**: Preheat your grill to medium-high heat (about 400°F or 200°C). If using a grill pan, heat it over medium-high heat on the stovetop. Ensure that the grill grates are clean and lightly oiled to prevent sticking. Preheating is crucial for achieving the perfect char and tenderness.

4. **Grill the Asparagus**: Once the grill is hot, place the asparagus spears perpendicular to the grates. This prevents them from falling through the gaps. Grill the asparagus for about 6-8 minutes, turning occasionally to ensure even cooking. You want the spears to be tender and slightly charred, with a vibrant green color.

5. **Season and Serve**: After grilling, remove the asparagus from the grill and transfer it to a serving platter. Season with salt and pepper to taste, adjusting the seasoning according to your preference. If desired, sprinkle grated Parmesan cheese over the asparagus for an added savory touch.

6. **Garnish**: For an extra burst of flavor and presentation, garnish the grilled asparagus with additional lemon zest or lemon wedges. The lemon wedges can be squeezed over the asparagus just before eating to enhance the citrusy flavor. This adds a refreshing element to the dish.

7. **Enjoy**: Serve the Grilled Asparagus with Lemon Zest warm as a side dish or incorporate it into a salad or grain bowl. This versatile dish pairs beautifully with grilled chicken, fish, or as part of a vegetarian meal. Enjoy the combination of flavors and the vibrant, fresh taste of the asparagus.

Nutritional Value (per serving, approximately 1 cup)

- **Calories**: ~70
- **Protein**: 3g
- **Carbohydrates**: 8g
- **Fiber**: 4g
- **Fat**: 4g
- **Saturated Fat**: 0.5g
- **Sugar**: 2g (naturally occurring)
- **Sodium**: 250mg (varies based on added salt)
- **Vitamin A**: 20% of daily recommended intake
- **Vitamin C**: 15% of daily recommended intake
- **Vitamin K**: 50% of daily recommended intake
- **Folate**: 10% of daily recommended intake
- **Iron**: 10% of daily recommended intake

Grilled Asparagus with Lemon Zest is not only a delicious addition to your meals but also a powerhouse of nutrition. Asparagus is low in calories and high in essential vitamins and minerals, making it an excellent choice for weight management and overall health. The healthy fats from olive oil aid in the absorption of fat-soluble vitamins, while lemon adds a refreshing flavor and boosts vitamin C content. This dish is quick to prepare, making it a perfect choice for busy weeknight dinners or elegant gatherings. Whether enjoyed on its own or as a side dish, grilled asparagus is a versatile and healthy addition to any anti-inflammatory diet.

Cauliflower Rice with Herbs and Lemon is a light, nutritious, and versatile dish that serves as a fantastic low-carb alternative to traditional rice. This dish harnesses the subtle, nutty flavor of cauliflower and pairs it with fresh herbs and zesty lemon, making it a refreshing side or a base for a variety of meals. Cauliflower is rich in vitamins C and K, as well as fiber, making it a great addition to an anti-inflammatory diet. The herbs not only enhance the flavor but also add their own health benefits, while the lemon juice provides a bright acidity that ties everything together. This dish is perfect for anyone looking to incorporate more vegetables into their diet while enjoying a satisfying and flavorful accompaniment to their main dishes.

Preparation Time

- **Prep Time**: 10 minutes
- **Cook Time**: 10 minutes
- **Total Time**: 20 minutes

Ingredients

- 1 medium head of cauliflower, trimmed and chopped into florets
- 2 tablespoons olive oil
- 1/4 cup onion, finely chopped
- 2 cloves garlic, minced
- Zest of 1 lemon
- 2 tablespoons fresh lemon juice
- 1/4 cup fresh parsley, chopped
- 2 tablespoons fresh basil, chopped
- Salt and pepper to taste
- Optional: 1/4 teaspoon red pepper flakes (for a spicy kick)

Procedure

1. **Prepare the Cauliflower**: Start by washing and trimming the cauliflower head, removing the leaves and stems. Cut it into small florets for easier processing. Using a food processor, pulse the florets in batches until they resemble rice grains in size and texture. Alternatively, you can grate the cauliflower using a box grater for a more hands-on approach. Ensure that you don't over-process it, as you want to maintain some texture.

2. **Sauté the Aromatics**: In a large skillet, heat 2 tablespoons of olive oil over medium heat. Add the finely chopped onion and sauté for 3-4 minutes, or until the onion becomes translucent and fragrant. Then, add the minced garlic and sauté for an additional minute, stirring constantly to prevent the garlic from burning. This step builds a flavorful base for the cauliflower rice.

3. **Cook the Cauliflower Rice**: Once the onions and garlic are ready, add the riced cauliflower to the skillet. Stir well to combine with the onion and garlic mixture. Cook for about 5-7 minutes, stirring occasionally, until the cauliflower is tender but still slightly crisp. Season with salt, pepper, and red pepper flakes (if using) to enhance the flavor.

4. **Add Lemon Zest and Juice**: After the cauliflower is cooked, remove the skillet from the heat. Stir in the lemon zest and fresh lemon juice, ensuring that the citrus flavors are evenly distributed throughout the cauliflower rice. This addition brightens the dish and gives it a refreshing zing that complements the cauliflower beautifully.

5. **Mix in Fresh Herbs**: Gently fold in the chopped parsley and basil, allowing the herbs to wilt slightly from the residual heat. The fresh herbs add a burst of flavor and a pop of color to the dish, making it visually appealing as well as delicious.

6. **Adjust Seasoning**: Taste the cauliflower rice and adjust the seasoning if necessary, adding more salt, pepper, or lemon juice to suit your preference. This step ensures that the flavors are balanced and to your liking.

7. **Serve**: Transfer the Cauliflower Rice with Herbs and Lemon to a serving dish and enjoy it warm. It makes a fantastic side dish for grilled meats, fish, or roasted vegetables, or can be served as a base for a grain bowl topped with your favorite protein and veggies. This dish is not only nutritious but also incredibly versatile and easy to customize with your favorite herbs or additional toppings.

Nutritional Value (per serving, approximately 1 cup)

- **Calories**: ~60
- **Protein**: 2g
- **Carbohydrates**: 4g
- **Fiber**: 2g
- **Fat**: 5g
- **Saturated Fat**: 0.5g
- **Sugar**: 2g (naturally occurring)
- **Sodium**: 150mg (varies based on added salt)
- **Vitamin C**: 75% of daily recommended intake
- **Vitamin K**: 15% of daily recommended intake
- **Folate**: 14% of daily recommended intake
- **Calcium**: 3% of daily recommended intake
- **Iron**: 4% of daily recommended intake

Cauliflower Rice with Herbs and Lemon is a flavorful and nutritious dish that can easily fit into various dietary preferences, including vegan, gluten-free, and low-carb diets. Cauliflower provides an excellent source of vitamins and minerals while being low in calories, making it a perfect option for weight management. The healthy fats from olive oil contribute to the absorption of fat-soluble vitamins, while the herbs and lemon enhance the dish's flavor profile. This recipe is quick to prepare, making it an ideal choice for busy weeknights or as part of meal prep. Enjoy the vibrant flavors and health benefits of this simple yet satisfying dish!

Sautéed Spinach with Garlic and Lemon is a quick and nutritious side dish that highlights the vibrant flavors of fresh spinach paired with aromatic garlic and zesty lemon. This dish not only provides a delicious accompaniment to a variety of meals but also boasts numerous health benefits due to the nutrient-dense nature of spinach. Packed with vitamins A, C, and K, as well as iron and antioxidants, sautéed spinach is an excellent addition to any anti-inflammatory diet. The garlic enhances the flavor while also offering its own health benefits, including potential anti-inflammatory properties. The brightness of the lemon juice lifts the dish and adds a refreshing twist that complements the earthiness of the spinach beautifully.

Preparation Time

- **Prep Time**: 5 minutes
- **Cook Time**: 5 minutes
- **Total Time**: 10 minutes

Ingredients

- 1 pound fresh spinach, washed and trimmed
- 2 tablespoons olive oil
- 3 cloves garlic, minced
- Zest of 1 lemon
- 2 tablespoons fresh lemon juice
- Salt and pepper to taste
- Optional: Red pepper flakes for a spicy kick

Procedure

1. **Prepare the Spinach**: Start by thoroughly washing the fresh spinach under cold water to remove any dirt or grit. Trim the stems if necessary and set aside to drain while you prepare the other ingredients. Using fresh spinach ensures a vibrant color and better flavor compared to pre-packaged varieties.

2. **Heat the Oil**: In a large skillet, heat 2 tablespoons of olive oil over medium heat. Allow the oil to warm for a minute; this will help the spinach cook evenly and impart its flavor. Olive oil not only adds a rich taste but also provides healthy fats that enhance nutrient absorption.

3. **Sauté the Garlic**: Once the oil is hot, add the minced garlic to the skillet. Sauté for about 30 seconds, stirring frequently to prevent burning. The garlic should become fragrant and slightly golden; be careful not to overcook it, as burnt garlic can taste bitter.

4. **Add the Spinach**: Add the washed spinach to the skillet, tossing it gently to coat with the garlic and olive oil. The spinach will begin to wilt quickly; continue to sauté for about 2-3 minutes until all the spinach is tender and bright green. Stirring ensures even cooking and prevents the leaves from sticking to the pan.

5. **Season and Flavor**: Once the spinach is cooked down, add the lemon zest and lemon juice to the skillet. Stir well to incorporate the citrus flavors throughout the spinach. Season with salt, pepper, and optional red pepper flakes for a touch of heat, adjusting to your taste preferences.

6. **Finish Cooking**: Allow the mixture to cook for an additional minute to let the flavors meld. The heat from the sautéed spinach will bring out the zestiness of the lemon and enhance the overall taste of the dish. Make sure not to overcook the spinach; it should retain a vibrant green color and slight crunch.

7. **Serve Immediately**: Remove the skillet from the heat and transfer the sautéed spinach to a serving dish. This dish is best enjoyed warm as a side to grilled proteins, fish, or even as a topping for grain bowls. The vibrant colors and fresh flavors make it a visually appealing and nutritious addition to any meal.

Nutritional Value (per serving, approximately 1 cup)

- **Calories**: ~50
- **Protein**: 3g
- **Carbohydrates**: 5g
- **Fiber**: 3g
- **Fat**: 4g
- **Saturated Fat**: 0.5g
- **Sugar**: 1g (naturally occurring)

- **Sodium**: 150mg (varies based on added salt)
- **Vitamin A**: 180% of daily recommended intake
- **Vitamin C**: 35% of daily recommended intake
- **Vitamin K**: 450% of daily recommended intake
- **Iron**: 15% of daily recommended intake
- **Calcium**: 10% of daily recommended intake

Sautéed Spinach with Garlic and Lemon is a wonderfully nutritious dish that can elevate any meal. Its quick preparation time makes it ideal for busy weeknights, while the flavors are sophisticated enough for entertaining guests. The combination of garlic and lemon not only enhances the taste but also maximizes the health benefits of the dish. Spinach is particularly beneficial for promoting healthy skin, vision, and bone health, thanks to its high levels of antioxidants and essential vitamins. This versatile recipe can also be easily adapted; consider adding other ingredients like pine nuts, feta cheese, or even sautéed mushrooms for a different twist. Enjoy this simple yet delicious dish as part of your anti-inflammatory diet!

30-Day Anti-Inflammatory Meal Plan

- **Day 1**
    - Breakfast: Flaxseed Banana Pancakes
    - Lunch: Quinoa Porridge with Cinnamon and Berries
    - Snack: Crispy Kale Chips with Nutritional Yeast
    - Dinner: Sweet Potato & Kale Breakfast Hash
- **Day 2**
    - Breakfast: Golden Glow Smoothie (Mango, Ginger, Turmeric)
    - Lunch: Quinoa and Arugula Salad with Lemon Vinaigrette
    - Snack: Cucumber Hummus Bites
    - Dinner: Baked Cod with Lemon, Garlic & Olive Oil
- **Day 3**
    - Breakfast: Avocado Toast with Hemp Seeds & Microgreens
    - Lunch: Anti-Inflammatory Power Bowl (Beets, Lentils, Kale)
    - Snack: Walnut & Berry Energy Bites
    - Dinner: Sweet Potato and Chickpea Curry
- **Day 4**
    - Breakfast: Blueberry Chia Pudding
    - Lunch: Roasted Sweet Potato & Spinach Salad
    - Snack: Turmeric Roasted Chickpeas
    - Dinner: Sautéed Tempeh with Ginger and Sesame
- **Day 5**
    - Breakfast: Anti-Inflammatory Green Smoothie
    - Lunch: Watermelon and Feta Anti-Inflammatory Salad
    - Snack: Avocado-Stuffed Bell Peppers
    - Dinner: Grilled Chicken with Avocado Salsa
- **Day 6**
    - Breakfast: Quinoa Porridge with Cinnamon and Berries
    - Lunch: Cucumber and Tomato Salad with Avocado & Basil
    - Snack: Ginger Garlic Green Beans
    - Dinner: Roasted Cauliflower Tacos with Spicy Yogurt Sauce
- **Day 7**
    - Breakfast: Golden Milk Smoothie Bowl
    - Lunch: Mango and Avocado Salad with Lime Dressing
    - Snack: Walnut & Berry Energy Bites
    - Dinner: Hearty Lentil and Vegetable Stew

- **Day 8**
    - o Breakfast: Flaxseed Banana Pancakes
    - o Lunch: Broccoli & Pomegranate Detox Salad
    - o Snack: Crispy Kale Chips with Nutritional Yeast
    - o Dinner: Turmeric Butternut Squash Soup
- **Day 9**
    - o Breakfast: Anti-Inflammatory Green Smoothie
    - o Lunch: Chickpea and Turmeric Couscous Salad
    - o Snack: Cucumber Hummus Bites
    - o Dinner: Sautéed Spinach with Garlic and Lemon
- **Day 10**
    - o Breakfast: Avocado Toast with Hemp Seeds & Microgreens
    - o Lunch: Zucchini Noodles with Pesto and Cherry Tomatoes
    - o Snack: Roasted Beetroot with Thyme
    - o Dinner: Grilled Asparagus with Lemon Zest
- **Day 11**
    - o Breakfast: Blueberry Chia Pudding
    - o Lunch: Quinoa Pilaf with Toasted Almonds and Cranberries
    - o Snack: Walnut & Berry Energy Bites
    - o Dinner: Spicy Black Bean Soup
- **Day 12**
    - o Breakfast: Golden Glow Smoothie
    - o Lunch: Roasted Brussels Sprouts with Balsamic Glaze
    - o Snack: Avocado-Stuffed Bell Peppers
    - o Dinner: Coconut and Matcha Protein Bars
- **Day 13**
    - o Breakfast: Flaxseed Banana Pancakes
    - o Lunch: Quinoa-Stuffed Bell Peppers
    - o Snack: Turmeric Roasted Chickpeas
    - o Dinner: Mushroom and Barley Soup
- **Day 14**
    - o Breakfast: Golden Milk Smoothie Bowl
    - o Lunch: Anti-Inflammatory Power Bowl (Beets, Lentils, Kale)
    - o Snack: Ginger Garlic Green Beans
    - o Dinner: Roasted Cauliflower Tacos with Spicy Yogurt Sauce

- **Day 15**
  - Breakfast: Quinoa Porridge with Cinnamon and Berries
  - Lunch: Roasted Sweet Potato & Spinach Salad
  - Snack: Crispy Kale Chips with Nutritional Yeast
  - Dinner: Grilled Chicken with Avocado Salsa
- **Day 16**
  - Breakfast: Avocado Toast with Hemp Seeds & Microgreens
  - Lunch: Zucchini and Basil Soup
  - Snack: Cucumber Hummus Bites
  - Dinner: Sweet Potato and Chickpea Curry
- **Day 17**
  - Breakfast: Flaxseed Banana Pancakes
  - Lunch: Mango and Avocado Salad with Lime Dressing
  - Snack: Roasted Beetroot with Thyme
  - Dinner: Sautéed Tempeh with Ginger and Sesame
- **Day 18**
  - Breakfast: Anti-Inflammatory Green Smoothie
  - Lunch: Broccoli & Pomegranate Detox Salad
  - Snack: Avocado-Stuffed Bell Peppers
  - Dinner: Hearty Lentil and Vegetable Stew
- **Day 19**
  - Breakfast: Golden Glow Smoothie
  - Lunch: Watermelon and Feta Anti-Inflammatory Salad
  - Snack: Walnut & Berry Energy Bites
  - Dinner: Turmeric Butternut Squash Soup
- **Day 20**
  - Breakfast: Golden Milk Smoothie Bowl
  - Lunch: Cucumber and Tomato Salad with Avocado & Basil
  - Snack: Ginger Garlic Green Beans
  - Dinner: Roasted Cauliflower Tacos with Spicy Yogurt Sauce
- **Day 21**
  - Breakfast: Blueberry Chia Pudding
  - Lunch: Quinoa and Arugula Salad with Lemon Vinaigrette
  - Snack: Crispy Kale Chips with Nutritional Yeast
  - Dinner: Sautéed Spinach with Garlic and Lemon

- **Day 22**
    - Breakfast: Flaxseed Banana Pancakes
    - Lunch: Chickpea and Turmeric Couscous Salad
    - Snack: Turmeric Roasted Chickpeas
    - Dinner: Grilled Chicken with Avocado Salsa
- **Day 23**
    - Breakfast: Quinoa Porridge with Cinnamon and Berries
    - Lunch: Zucchini Noodles with Pesto and Cherry Tomatoes
    - Snack: Walnut & Berry Energy Bites
    - Dinner: Mushroom and Barley Soup
- **Day 24**
    - Breakfast: Golden Milk Smoothie Bowl
    - Lunch: Roasted Sweet Potato & Spinach Salad
    - Snack: Avocado-Stuffed Bell Peppers
    - Dinner: Spicy Black Bean Soup
- **Day 25**
    - Breakfast: Anti-Inflammatory Green Smoothie
    - Lunch: Quinoa Pilaf with Toasted Almonds and Cranberries
    - Snack: Cucumber Hummus Bites
    - Dinner: Coconut and Matcha Protein Bars
- **Day 26**
    - Breakfast: Blueberry Chia Pudding
    - Lunch: Anti-Inflammatory Power Bowl (Beets, Lentils, Kale)
    - Snack: Ginger Garlic Green Beans
    - Dinner: Grilled Asparagus with Lemon Zest
- **Day 27**
    - Breakfast: Golden Glow Smoothie
    - Lunch: Quinoa-Stuffed Bell Peppers
    - Snack: Roasted Beetroot with Thyme
    - Dinner: Turmeric Butternut Squash Soup
- **Day 28**
    - Breakfast: Flaxseed Banana Pancakes
    - Lunch: Cucumber and Tomato Salad with Avocado & Basil
    - Snack: Crispy Kale Chips with Nutritional Yeast
    - Dinner: Sweet Potato and Chickpea Curry

- **Day 29**
    - o Breakfast: Avocado Toast with Hemp Seeds & Microgreens
    - o Lunch: Broccoli & Pomegranate Detox Salad
    - o Snack: Walnut & Berry Energy Bites
    - o Dinner: Grilled Chicken with Avocado Salsa
- **Day 30**
    - o Breakfast: Golden Milk Smoothie Bowl
    - o Lunch: Zucchini and Basil Soup
    - o Snack: Turmeric Roasted Chickpeas
    - o Dinner: Baked Cod with Lemon, Garlic & Olive Oil

This meal plan ensures you enjoy a wide range of nutrient-dense, anti-inflammatory meals each day, promoting good digestion, reduced inflammation, and balanced energy levels for the month.

Conclusion

Congratulations on making it through the *Flat Belly Anti-Inflammatory Diet for Beginners 2025!* By now, you've equipped yourself with a treasure trove of delicious recipes that not only promote health but also celebrate the joy of eating. Who knew that a plateful of vibrant veggies could pack such a punch, both in taste and in the fight against inflammation?

As you embark on this culinary journey, remember that healthy eating doesn't mean sacrificing flavor. It means embracing a lifestyle where nutritious choices are just as delightful as your favorite comfort foods—without the post-meal food coma. And let's face it, no one enjoys a heavy stomach while lounging on the couch binge-watching their favorite show!

So whether you're whipping up a *Turmeric Roasted Chickpea* or indulging in a *Sweet Potato and Chickpea Curry*, know that you're not just feeding your body but also treating your taste buds to a fiesta of flavors. Keep experimenting, keep exploring, and keep smiling!

Remember, your kitchen is your laboratory, and each recipe is an experiment in deliciousness. Who knows? You might just invent the next viral dish that sends everyone into a food frenzy! So go ahead, grab those veggies, channel your inner chef, and don't forget to share your tasty triumphs (and maybe even a few culinary blunders) with your friends. After all, laughter and good food are the best ingredients for a happy life!

Here's to your health, happiness, and the countless adventures awaiting you in the world of anti-inflammatory cooking. Cheers!

www.ingramcontent.com/pod-product-compliance
Lightning Source LLC
Chambersburg PA
CBHW081213260726
48653CB00010BA/3635